SLEEPING WITH YOUR BABY: A PARENT'S GUIDE TO COSLEEPING

James J. McKenna, Ph.D.

Platypus Media®, LLC
Washington, DC

Copyright 2007 Platypus Media®, LLC
First edition • May 2007
ISBN: 1-930775-34-2 / ISBN-13: 978-1-930775-34-3

This book is not intended to be a replacement for advice from your health care provider. An important part of informed self-care is knowing when to seek out your community's health care resources. Readers should consult a physician or professional health care provider on a regular basis. This book is not meant to be a substitute for your doctor. It is a general informational guide and reference source. No medical or legal responsibility is assumed by the author or publisher.

Published in the United States by:
Platypus Media®, LLC
627 A Street, NE
Washington, DC 20002
Toll-free: 877-PLATYPS (877-872-8977) or 202-546-1674
Fax: 202-546-2356
www.PlatypusMedia.com
Info@PlatypusMedia.com

Distributed to the book trade in the United States by:
National Book Network
Toll Free 800-787-6859 / 301-459-3366 / Fax 301-429-5746
CustServ@nbnbooks.com / www.nbnbooks.com

Library of Congress Cataloging-in-Publication Data
McKenna, James J. (James Joseph), 1948-
Sleeping with your baby : a parent's guide to cosleeping / James J. McKenna. — 1st ed.
p. cm.
Includes index.
ISBN-13: 978-1-930775-34-3
ISBN-10: 1-930775-34-2
1. Co-sleeping. I. Title.
GT3000.5.C67M35 2007
649'.122—dc22
2006031063

10 9 8 7 6 5 4 3 2 1

Manufactured in the United States of America

WHAT THE EXPERTS

"I am delighted to endorse this excellent guide for parents. It provides masses of information to help new parents make informed choices on whether to cosleep or bedshare with their baby, how to do so safely, and when bedsharing should be avoided. It also answers all those questions about bedsharing that parents often ask, such as how long bedsharing might continue, how it affects a child's development, cobedding of twins, and whether it is safe to sleep with a premature baby. The appendices and bibliography provide valuable resources for parents wishing to explore these issues further. This book will help parents and health professionals alike to understand and discuss the issues regarding bedsharing, and to make thoughtful choices."

Helen Ball, Ph.D., BSc, MA
Senior Lecturer in Anthropology & Director
Parent-Infant Sleep Lab
Durham University, UK

"Cosleeping is one of the most delicious experiences in parenting, and Dr. McKenna's carefully researched and thoughtful advice separates the myths from the marvelous reality."

Harvey Karp, M.D.
Assistant Professor of Pediatrics
UCLA School of Medicine
Author of the book/DVD *The Happiest Baby on the Block*

"Jim McKenna's new book, *Sleeping with Your Baby,* is a wonderfully readable volume filled with excellent science and clear, safe, sensible guidance for parents by a real expert who has spent his life studying infant sleep. The introductory chapter, entitled "Why I Care So Much About This Subject" is, by itself, worth the price of the book. But do read the whole book."

Lawrence M. Gartner, M.D.
Professor Emeritus
Departments of Pediatrics and Obstetrics/Gynecology
The University of Chicago

"Jim McKenna has provided us with sound advice, based on the best current evidence, on the best options for the safest sleeping settings. Thank you, Dr. McKenna, for providing every parent with food for thought, based on a multidisciplinary assessment of the literature, and for offering recommendations for every safe sleeping setting."

Miriam H. Labbok, M.D., MPH, FACPM, IBCLC, FABM
Director, Center for Infant and Young Child Feeding and Care
University of North Carolina—Chapel Hill

"Brilliant! Finally a book on sleep written by a research scientist who has spent much of his academic career studying bedsharing and its relationship to maternal and child health. This information is vital to all who care about infants, parenting issues, public health issues—both mental and physical—and our society in general. One of my proudest achievements is that I "discovered" Jim McKenna in 1989 and introduced him to both the professional and mother support breastfeeding worlds. Now it is with great pride that I recommend this book to the breastfeeding world and the world at large."

> Chele Marmet, MA, IBCLC
> Director
> Lactation Institute
> Conceptualized and pioneered the field of lactation

"Dr. McKenna clearly differentiates cultural bias from science in a very balanced and readable way, so that parents are empowered to make the correct choices for themselves regarding safe bedsharing and cosleeping."

> Nancy E. Wight, M.D., IBCLC, FABM, FAAP
> Medical Director, Lactation Services
> Sharp Mary Birch Hospital for Women

"Dr. James McKenna offers parents a comprehensive well-researched look at cosleeping and its vital benefits to the infant on all developmental levels. To ensure the safe practice of cosleeping, Dr. McKenna carefully explores the myths and the facts providing parents with evidence and practical guidelines for its normal, natural practice. I am grateful for this valuable and timely guide and I will actively present this all-inclusive resource to parents internationally."

> Jeanne Ohm, D.C.
> Executive Coordinator
> International Chiropractic Pediatric Association

"BRAVO! Jim McKenna's book *Sleeping with Your Baby: A Parent's Guide to Cosleeping* is a fabulous resource, and very much needed! Dr. McKenna deftly analyzes decades of research in human biology, sleep physiology, and anthropology and merges the best of science with practical, comfortable, and safety-conscious guidelines for parents and professionals."

> Linda J. Smith, BSE, FACCE, IBCLC
> Bright Future Lactation Resource Centre, Ltd.

Agencies, organizations and individuals interested in purchasing multiple copies of this book can receive a bulk discount for quantity orders. Please contact us at:

Platypus Media®, LLC
627 A Street, NE
Washington, DC 20002
Toll-free: 877-PLATYPS (877-872-8977)
202-546-1674
Fax: 202-546-2356
www.PlatypusMedia.com
Info@PlatypusMedia.com

Senior Editor: Tracey Kilby, Washington, DC
Editor: Amy Condra, Macon, GA
Proofreading: Katherine M. Isaacs, Montpelier, VT
Designer: Doug Wink, Inkway Graphics, Santa Fe, NM
Cover Design: Andrew Barthelmes, Peekskill, NY

USBC statement, reprinted with permission.
ILCA statement, reprinted with permission.
LLLI statement, reprinted with permission.

Photo credits:
Pages 23, 25, 35, 38, 48, 51, 53, 59, 64, 65, 75, 77, 79, 81, 90, 91, 92, 93, 94, 95, 96, 97   Photos from www.dreamstime.com
Pages 30, 86   Photos courtesy of Ms. Molly Pesse, Evergreen Hospital
Page 33   Photo courtesy of Robert Copeland, Mark-It Television
Pages 42, 83, 89   Photos courtesy of Rosie Moyer, www.littlelaughs.com
Page 61   Photo courtesy of Sabrina Raheem
Page 66   Photos courtesy of the Consumer Product Safety Commission
Page 67   Photo courtesy of James McKenna
Page 69   Illustration by Andrew Barthelmes
Pages 72, 73   Photos courtesy of Arm's Reach®
Page 84   Photo by Lucille Weinstat

his book is designed to describe the present scientific status and medical and social controversies in the field of cosleeping, and why there is no consensus on the issue of bedsharing. It is intended to educate parents about safe and unsafe sleeping environments according to all lines of scientific evidence, and to let parents of healthy, full-term infants know how to best avoid recognized adverse conditions that can make forms of cosleeping and bedsharing dangerous. This book is not intended to advocate any one form of sleeping arrangement, but to clarify the importance of matching the best sleeping arrangement to each particular family, and to inform parents about the potential benefits of sleeping close to baby where and when safe conditions can be met.

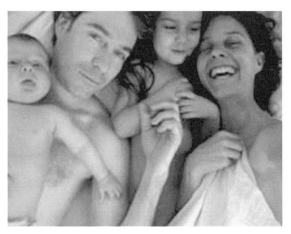

Many children are less physically and emotionally healthy than they could be. The current epidemic of childhood obesity suggests that children are overfed but probably undernourished... What is a successful child? A child who's happy, well adjusted, and morally grounded... a successful child is an attached child — connected not just to family, but to the world beyond.

William Sears, MD and Martha Sears, RN
The Successful Child

This book is dedicated to my mother, Mary Virginia Lane McKenna,
who managed to raise six children without ever consulting Dr. Spock;
and to the loving memory of Grant Elsberry and his parents Dan and Lisa,
who know both the height of love and the depth of loss.

TABLE OF CONTENTS

PREFACE

Meredith Small, Ph.D.

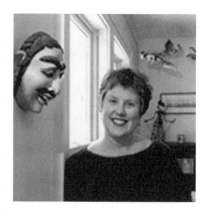

You can trust Jim McKenna. You can especially trust what he says about cosleeping because Jim is an honest, thoughtful person, and even more importantly, his advice on infant-parent sleep is based on science, history, anthropology, and a thorough knowledge of human evolution. His advice is also informed by what is biologically and emotionally best for babies and parents and how attachments form and grow. And he has practical experience with cosleeping; Jim is a father, with a grown son who turned out great (and with whom he coslept).

You can also trust Jim because he has stayed the course in advocating cosleeping, even during the worst storms of what has become a major controversy, especially in America—what a surprising place for an academic such as Jim. Scholars usually stick to their lab and field sites, working on esoteric bits of knowledge up in an Ivory Tower where the public pays them no mind. But ever since Jim first became intrigued by infant sleep, he has doggedly pursued the issue and tirelessly talked to the public about how our culture has misconstrued what babies really need. He has, in a sense, set out to change our culture, and in that quest, he has become not just an observer of human behavior, but one who wants to change behavior for the better. That is no easy feat.

All cultures hold their values dear. Most often, those values are so much a part of daily life that they are not even recognized until some revolutionary citizen decides to behave in a way that differs from the current norm. Or until some anthropologist comes along and points out that people in other cultures have different ideas and that there might be any number of kinds of "normal." Where babies sleep is such a controversial issue in Western culture because it is embedded (no pun intended) in our ideology of fostering independence in all our citizens, even babies. We may talk about the importance of family, but in Western culture, the point is to be off alone, making decisions alone, and getting through the emotional storm of life alone, needing no one. Our fear of sharing a bed with a baby is also tainted by the accepted pattern of daily life in Western culture. One "should" work all day, be with family in the evening and on weekends, and sleep alone (oddly, adults are allowed to cosleep, but only with other adults), deeply and through the night. The bed in the West is also synonymous with sex, and that, too, makes cosleeping with an infant suspect.

But Jim McKenna has taken on all these culturally held beliefs and turned them upside down. He has done this by being a good scientist. His sleep lab work demonstrates the nocturnal connection between a baby and a parent by tracking physiological changes in both sleepers and visuals of their nighttime tango. That connection, as Jim has shown, is biologically based and measurable. He has also researched where babies sleep in many other cultures, and followed the path of sleeping traditions through history in Western culture to understand why in the world we are now so adamant, and so righteous, about where babies sleep. Based on all of this knowledge, McKenna recommends cosleeping, as long as it's under safe conditions, because it's best for babies and parents. You can trust this advice because Jim has looked at this issue from every single possible angle.

The accepted norm in Western culture is singular sleep for babies; this is what the pediatricians recommend and what the grandparents expect. And so cosleeping has become a revolutionary act. But parents who choose to cosleep with their infants don't feel like revolutionaries, they just want to stay close to their babies. Thank goodness we have Jim to assure cosleeping families that their choice is normal and natural, no matter what the culture says.

Trust Jim McKenna, and sleep tight.

Dr. Meredith Small, author of *Our Babies, Ourselves; How Biology and Culture Shape the Way We Parent* and *Kids: How Biology and Culture Shape the Way We Raise Young Children* is a professor of anthropology at Cornell University. Trained as a primate behaviorist, she is now interested in the intersection of biology and culture and how that intersection affects the health and well being of children. Small also writes for the popular audience and is a commentator on NPR's *All Things Considered.*

FOREWORD

Peter Fleming, M.D., Ph.D.

For most human beings, through most of human history, the question of where and with whom a baby should sleep would simply not have been asked. The importance of close mother-infant contact and accessibility of the mother for breastfeeding was so central to infant survival that to suggest any alternative would have been seen as tantamount to neglect or abuse.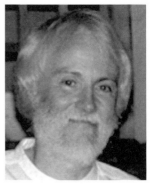
In the late 19th century, a number of investigators, trying to unravel the mystery of apparently increasing numbers of infants dying in the poorer quarters of great cities (particularly London) came to the conclusion that because most of these deaths occurred in bed with parents, the deaths were a direct consequence of being in bed with parents—compounded by recognized contributions from heavy parental alcohol use and overall poverty. Over 100 years later, the American Academy of Pediatrics came to similar conclusions, based upon extrapolation of carefully collected data on the interaction of various risk factors and mother-infant bedsharing.

Professor McKenna's book seeks to clarify the apparent conflict between the anthropological literature—which emphasizes the value and importance of mother-infant interactions in facilitating and directing infant development—and pediatric literature—which focuses on the potential hazards of bedsharing as a risk factor for unexpected infant deaths. The reality, as elegantly shown by Dr. McKenna, is that there is no conflict—merely a different way of looking at the same information.

This helpful exposition of the importance of mother-infant contact throughout the 24 hours of the infant's day also makes it quite clear that, in certain circumstances and for certain individuals, sharing a sleep surface may be hazardous for infants. It also shows, however, that provided parents are aware of the potential risks as well as the potential benefits, and are able to eliminate identifiable hazards, then bedsharing—or at the very least mothers and infants sleeping in close proxim-

13

ity even if not sharing a surface—can be both safe and fulfilling for mothers and babies.

The information contained within this book should be compulsory core knowledge for those caring for parents and infants in whatever capacity. It exemplifies the importance of not letting rare and potentially avoidable tragedies distort our understanding of how we all grew and developed as infants. When it comes to making decisions about child care, there is no substitute for a well-informed parent.

Dr. Peter J. Fleming, after qualifying in medicine in 1972 and gaining a Ph.D. in physiology, plus specialist qualifications in both adult medicine and pediatrics, has worked in the fields of newborn and infant care and children's sleep medicine for almost 30 years. As head of the research team in Avon that identified many of the risk factors for Sudden Infant Death Syndrome (SIDS), he led the implementation of the "Back to Sleep" campaigns in the UK and several other countries in the early 1990s, and has continued his research in this area, with a particular emphasis on the effects of mother-infant interactions and the effects of infant sleep environments. His greatest sources of knowledge and inspiration in this (and every other) field are Jo, his wife (a family doctor), and their four wonderful sons.

INTRODUCTION

William Sears, M.D.

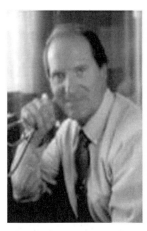

In 1978 our adventures of sleeping with our babies began. Prior to that year, our first three children were easy sleepers and we were part of the crib-and-cradle set. Then came our fourth child, Hayden, whose birth changed our parenting night life forever. As we had with our previous children, we customarily placed Hayden in her crib in the early weeks, but she awoke frequently, as if experiencing a sort of nighttime anxiety. One night my exhausted wife, Martha, said, "I don't care what the books say. I've got to get some sleep..." She welcomed Hayden into our bed, the nursing pair slept peacefully, and the rest is beautiful history.

We coslept with our next four infants—one at a time—until weaning. As a young pediatrician with no medical training in where babies should sleep I was fascinated by the restful synchrony that I saw between the nursing pair. Martha would partially awaken just before Hayden would. Martha would nurse or comfort her back to sleep and neither member of the nursing pair completely awakened. Wow! Something good is happening here, I thought. If only I could wire up mother and baby and scientifically prove that something healthful is going on between them when they share a bed, then I could quiet the separate-sleeping crowd who warned us of the "bad habit," saying "she'll never get out of your bed," and the unwarranted fears of terminal dependency. The prevailing nighttime mindset of the time was fostering self-soothing and early independence.

Then, in 1981, I met Dr. McKenna whose interest and passion was to scientifically study mothers and babies in various sleeping arrangements and to document the physiological differences between cosleepers and separate sleepers. I still remember at our lunch meeting saying, "Jim, I'm going to follow your studies very carefully, since I'm certain a lot of good things occur while mother and baby sleep close to each other. I just can't prove it." My medical motto has always been "show me the science." Childrearing is too valuable to be left to opinions alone. Besides, I was then dubbed, "The daring doctor who recommends mothers sleep with their babies."

Twenty-five years and many scientific articles later, Dr. McKenna has proved what intuitive parents have long suspected: something healthful happens to mother and baby when they cosleep. In this book, Dr. McKenna shows us the science. Readers can trust that Dr. McKenna's practical advice is backed up by his thousands of hours spent in the sleep laboratory monitoring sleep-sharing pairs, and he relates his observations in easy-to-read language and captivating conclusions.

In nighttime parenting our eight children, we learned a valuable lesson in deciding where babies should sleep: get behind the eyes of your baby and ask yourself, "If I were my baby, where would I want to sleep?" Would your baby want to sleep alone in a separate room, behind bars, with a high risk of experiencing nighttime anxiety, or would your baby rather be nestled next to their favorite person in the whole wide world and enjoy nighttime restfulness?

In this book you will find trusted advice from the world's authority on sleeping with your baby.

Dr. William Sears, or Dr. Bill as his 'little' patients call him, is the father of eight children as well as the author of over 30 books on childcare. He is an Associate Clinical Professor of Pediatrics at the University of California, Irvine, School of Medicine, and received his pediatric training at Harvard Medical School's Children's Hospital in Boston and The Hospital for Sick Children in Toronto. Dr. Sears is a fellow of the American Academy of Pediatrics (AAP) and a fellow of the Royal College of Pediatricians (RCP). He is also a medical and parenting consultant for *BabyTalk* and *Parenting* magazines and pediatrician for the website Parenting.com.

ABOUT THE AUTHOR

Professor James J. McKenna, Ph.D., is the Rev. Edmund P. Joyce C.S.C. Chair in Anthropology at the University of Notre Dame. He also directs the Mother-Baby Behavioral Sleep Laboratory at the University. He has published extensively on infant sleep, breastfeeding, Sudden Infant Death Syndrome (SIDS), and the evolution of human behavior, with special emphasis on the differences between the behavior and physiology of solitary, cosleeping and breastfeeding mother-baby pairs. His interests include how cultural factors influence infant and childcare practices, which, in turn, affect maternal-infant health and well-being. The National Institutes of Child Health and Human Development fund his research. Currently, he is involved in a multi-site U.S.A. national prospective project examining first-time teen moms throughout their pregnancies and throughout the first three years of their infants' lives. His articles have appeared in periodicals and academic journals around the world, and he is considered one of the leading authorities on scientific studies of infant-parent cosleeping and breastfeeding, especially bedsharing, having been the first to study the practice. He is a sought-after speaker for pediatric conferences and health, professional, parenting, and policy conferences around the globe. Visit his homepage at http://www.nd.edu/ ~ jmckenn1/lab.

WHY I CARE SO MUCH ABOUT THIS SUBJECT

James J. McKenna, Ph.D.

"There is no such thing as a baby, there is a baby and someone."

D.H. WINNICOTT

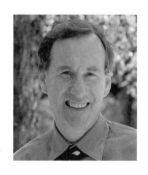

Many of my friends find it amusing that I spend almost all my waking hours studying what people do when they sleep. It is true. What people do when they are asleep fascinates me—and not just people in general, but families, in particular. As Director of the Mother-Baby Behavioral Sleep Laboratory at the University of Notre Dame, my students and I study, among other things, infant-parent cosleeping, nighttime breastfeeding, and especially bedsharing. The research is not just for the sake of gathering knowledge. It is for helping mothers and infants to sleep better, to thrive physically and emotionally, and even to save lives.

When it comes to parenting, new moms and dads are inundated by conflicting advice from relatives, well meaning friends, medical professionals, the media, the government and, of course, from other parents. The vast majority of parents want to do the best for their children, yet this bombardment of information certainly implies that parental wisdom and the capacity of parents to make their own informed decisions is somehow out of their grasp. It is as if everyone *else* knows exactly what is best for your baby.

Bedsharing, sleeping next to one's baby, and lying the infant on his back for sleep (which facilitates breastfeeding) is so universal and widespread, most parents worldwide couldn't imagine asking where their baby should sleep, whether it is it ok to sleep with the baby, what position the baby should sleep in and how the baby should be fed.

With the birth of our son, Jeffrey, in 1978, my wife Joanne and I entered the world of parenting. Anxious about our new set of responsibilities, we read book after book on parenting. We were both anthropologists, but were quite taken aback at what we found in the childcare literature. When it came to what the experts had to say about feeding patterns and sleeping arrangements, we were very confused. Either all our research and training about the universal aspects of human life were wrong, or the pediatric experts were missing or ignoring key information.

We learned that not only was there nothing in the childcare books that reflected anything about what we had learned about our primate heritage and sleeping arrangements, but nothing was reflected about what current neurobiological and psychological research was uncovering about human infant biology and the role of maternal touch in promoting human infant growth and well being. Further, we learned that infant care recommendations were not based on empirical laboratory or field studies of human infants at all, nor on cross-cultural insights as to how human babies actually lived.

Rather, they were based on 70 or 80 year old cultural ideas, uniquely Western and historically novel, mostly reflecting the social values of male physicians who not only had never changed a diaper, but had never—in any substantial way—associated with, or taken care of, their own infants. These were essentially middle-aged men who preferred to define babies in terms of who they wanted the infants to become, rather than in terms of who they actually were—little creatures who are very much dependent physiologically, socially, and psychologically on the presence of the caregiver to an unprecedented degree for an unprecedented length of time compared with other mammals.

The more we delved into these areas, the more we discovered that the prevailing wisdom had no basis in science whatsoever. This discovery changed my career.

Western social values heavily emphasize infant self-sufficiency as early in life as is possible for infants. This historical fact about our culture makes it is easier to understand why, without any scientists actually testing to see if it were true, it was assumed that early nighttime infant separation from the parents was necessary to produce happy, confident, emotionally healthy, independent future adults, alongside magnificently energized parents content to live nighttime lives separate from their babies and children. Without any anthropological studies which could have cast serious doubt on these assumptions, a separate sleep space along with controlled bottle feeding was promoted. Pediatricians and child care experts erroneously claimed that this promoted an infant's ability to "self-soothe" and would lead to infants becoming independent adults.

During the nineties at the University of California Irvine School of Medicine Sleep Disorders Laboratory, my colleagues Drs. Sarah Mosko, Chris Richards, Claibourne Dungy, Sean Drummond and I conducted the first research on the physiological and behavioral differences between solitary and bedsharing sleeping mothers and babies.[1] Two pilot studies and a larger three-year study began for the first time to document exclusively breastfeeding infants sleeping next to their mothers (which from a biological perspective amounts to normal human infant sleep patterns). Our work (funded by the National Institutes of Child Health and Human Development) was the first to explore how sleeping arrangements impact both the mothers' and the infants' nighttime physiology and behavior.[1] Nighttime behavioral studies have continued at the University of Notre Dame Mother-Baby Behavioral Sleep Laboratory, where we continue to clearly demonstrate the special abilities of low- and high-risk mothers to respond to their infants' needs while bedsharing.

It may appear that not much happens during an infant's sleep period, and that the infant's body simply requires downtime each day. This is not the case. During sleep, all manner of physical and neurological processes, including developing inter-connections between new cells, are taking place. During this time, the brain is sorting out how many and which brain cells (affecting intellectual, emotional and psychological aspects of development) will be retained rather than "pruned." The young brains of human infants need to reduce the nutrient demand of cells that don't seem to be used often so that nutrients can be shifted to those cells that are.

Without the stimulation from maternal-infant contact and interactions—including nighttime sensory exchanges—neonatal brain cells are potentially lost forever. This has led some developmental psychologists to argue that infants are far more threatened by what they do not receive in terms of neurological excitation than by what they do, since "pruned" infant brain cells are not retrievable at a later date. Minimal contact with mother's body can make the neurological scaffolding less stable and effective, weakening the structures that provide the basis of the infant's rapidly growing communicative skills, emotionality, and ability to effectively regulate and respond to its own needs.[2]

Generations of parents have been instructed to put the child to bed separate and alone, in order to both promote the child's independence and the adults' intimacy. This cultural legacy is ingrained in Western societies. Parents who sleep with their infants are often considered needy or deficient. When we hear about babies who do not or cannot sleep alone through the night, rarely do we hear: "What a good baby!" even though such contact is exactly what is in a human infant's biological best interest.

The good news is that just recently, and for the first time, the American Academy of Pediatrics (AAP) recommends that infants should sleep "proximate" to the mother in the same room. The bad news is that they argue against sleeping on the same surface, in the same bed. Herein lies the controversy.

This is why I wrote this book. I want to share with you what I (and others) have learned. I want families to understand how much happens during sleep and bedsharing, including communicating with each other through touch, scent, sound, and taste. This unconscious communication is part of the way our species has evolved to maximize health and survival, and it is likewise an intrinsic part of the way parents communicate and experience love for, and with, their infants and each other. A baby sleeping on its own, in a crib, outside the supervision and monitoring of its mother or father is deprived of this vital communication and is, as scientific studies prove, at risk.

When you look at the prevalence of cosleeping in the mammal world, and among different cultures and in different eras of human history, it is clear that cosleeping is universal through time, and is practiced far and wide and in many different ways. My own intuition told me that something this common had to be beneficial, but it has only been through extensive and rigorous scientific study that we have determined this to be the case. Cosleeping is not only normal, common and instinctive, but it can be in the best interest of the family when it is elected for purposes of protecting and nurturing infants, when safety is given a priority, and when the right kind of cosleeping is chosen by each unique family.

That being said, one cannot be naïve regarding the different ways in which people live. There is no guarantee that anything we do with infants is done necessarily in a safe way. Cosleeping in the form of bedsharing is no different. It is quite true that bedsharing can be practiced in ways that are very dangerous. Bedsharing is generally a more complex and less stable practice than is crib sleeping, which has both advantages and disadvantages for babies. The point is that we need to educate families to avoid bedsharing where known adverse bedsharing risks do exist. One-size-*does-not*-fit-all when it comes to sleeping arrangements. Being aware of where dangers lie and what can and cannot be modified is critical. Where households exhibit identifiable risk factors for dangerous bedsharing, we must encourage alternative sleep practices.

The truth is no sleep environment is completely risk free. But the fact that a bedsharing environment cannot be made 100 % risk free is no more an argument for a global recommendation against any and all bedsharing than it is an argument for a global recommendation against any and all crib sleeping (because crib sleeping incurs risks, too). Using a different example, consider that thousands of people die while eating (from choking) every year, even though eating is normal, common and instinctive. In order to minimize the risks, adults are not advised to stop eating but instead instructed to learn the Heimlich maneuver and parents are instructed in food preparation and feeding techniques for young children.

Similarly, we learn with great effort how to properly use and place infants in car seats, rather than banning automobile transportation for infants because many babies die each year in cars due to some parents' disregard for the ways to minimize car travel risks.

This book is intended to provide a balanced, comprehensive and holistic perspective on cosleeping and bedsharing, specifically while breastfeeding. It is intended to provide safety information and reassurance to those families who are considering, or who choose to, sleep with their babies. Enjoying every minute with your baby—whether you are awake or asleep—is important because our time with them is very short. I hope that this book will enable you to feel comfortable holding, carrying and responding to your baby, and will help you feel good about your care-giving choices. I know I am not alone in wanting to help you and your family thrive and enjoy experiences that will be cherished forever.

Jim McKenna
May 2007

PART I:

AN INTRODUCTION TO COSLEEPING

WHAT IS COSLEEPING?

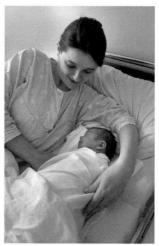

Many people don't fully understand the term "cosleeping," but they use the term nonetheless because most have a sense of what it is. Picture a mother lion and her cubs sleeping in a big heap, paws on top of backs, heads on bellies, body parts rising and falling with each rhythmic breath, the whole group intertwined in one peaceful lump of warmth and touching—that is cosleeping, or at least one version of it.

Of course, each species cosleeps uniquely in a manner reflecting the special biological needs and characteristics of its infants and mothers. For example, primates (including humans) typically give birth to one offspring at a time, providing each infant the opportunity to sleep alone with the mother or father. This way each infant can receive maximum attention during a very long and vulnerable infancy. Human infants are especially in need of a great deal of contact, emotional support, breastfeeding, and transportation.

Cosleeping refers to the many different ways babies sleep in close emotional and physical contact with their parents, usually within arms reach. Whether it is for protection, warmth, food, or comfort, humans and other mammals routinely sleep side by side, generation after generation. This book is about cosleeping, as practiced here in Western cultures and around the globe. In one way or another cosleeping remains universal for our species, predating history itself.

Cosleeping cannot necessarily be characterized the same way across all situations, but must be further broken down into safe and unsafe. And while each family's circumstances may vary, they can all be said to "cosleep" whenever they cuddle, snuggle and snooze together close enough to detect and respond to each other—whether on the same surface or not, and when at least one adult is committed to the infant's well being.

It is very important to acknowledge that cosleeping does not simply refer to bedsharing, for example, but it refers also to roomsharing, or any situation in which parents and infants are within arms' reach but not necessarily sleeping on the same surface. One of the difficult issues facing us is to reach agreement that while not all forms of cosleeping are safe, not all forms of cosleeping are dangerous, either. For example, some medical authorities mistakenly state that "cosleeping is dangerous," when they really mean to say that couch or sofa cosleeping is dangerous (which is always true) or, in their opinion, that bedsharing is dangerous (which may or may not be true, depending on how it is practiced). To speak about cosleeping without specifying what type of cosleeping one is referring to is to create more controversy and confusion than is necessary. While there may still be differences of opinion as to how to read the scientific findings on bedsharing (as I report below) there is generally much more agreement on some of these issues than it might appear.

There is no one right way to cosleep, nor does cosleeping occur in one correct configuration. While some ways of cosleeping are safer than other ways, some are not safe at all. One thing is for sure—regardless of whether or not you sleep on the same or a different surface, or in the same or a different room, remember that no one knows your baby better than you, and no one can anticipate and respond to the immediate needs of your baby as well as you. Families have shared sleep on futons, mats, mattresses, floors, and in hammocks. Around the world, parents continue to share sleep by having their babies within arms' reach—hanging in a swing attached to the roof, bundled up in a leather or cloth bag above them or in a camel-lined pouch, or attached to a cradle board.

Some cosleepers lie next to each other on the floor. Some Americans pull their bed frames apart to get rid of dangerous spaces between furniture parts and lay a mattress in the center of the room, away from walls—if a parent chooses to bedshare, this is likely the safest way to do it. Others sleep in the same room in close proximity to each other, with the adult on a bed and the baby in a bassinet or crib a few feet away. Still others fall asleep in individual rooms, and then come together in the middle of the night (when it is time for a feeding or someone has awoken and wants to change beds).

Cosleeping can be an ever-evolving process—babies may move from a crib, where they are placed at the beginning of the night, to their parent's bed, to a bassinet, and back again. My discussions with thousands of parents through the years tell me that there is generally not just one environment within which an infant sleeps, but several. Your baby may fall asleep in your bed and stay there all night, or may fall asleep in your bed and be moved later during sleep, or may fall asleep elsewhere and be welcomed in for a feeding in the middle of the night—or you may fall asleep in the baby's room and sleep some or all of the night there. Cosleeping can be practiced the same way, night after night, or can vary and shift as the baby grows and the adults' needs change.

All of this variability illustrates what parents of newborns quickly discover—their baby's sleep patterns are subject to frequent change, and sometimes it is hard to predict where exactly any given baby will sleep. As babies experience teething, they may have a difficult time sleeping. As newborns grow into older babies and toddlers, their cognitive and emotional development will affect their nighttime needs. As infants begin to place meaning on their daily experiences (some of them frightening), they might need more comforting to help them deal with increased confusion and nightmares. During times of stress, being close throughout the night is especially reassuring for your child. Bringing a baby into bed and nursing throughout the night are simple ways of meeting a child's needs, regardless of family income, educational background, or social status.

Sharing sleep with babies is natural for most families in non-industrialized cultures, but families in industrialized societies must often "relearn" specific methods of cosleeping. In other words, most of us have very little experience with cosleeping, as our own parents likely did not practice it and we are left unprepared.

It is true that we need to be very conscious of how we cosleep. If bedsharing, how we arrange bedding, other children, pets, and furniture must be done with care. In order to protect and promote the well-being of your baby, you will need to be aware of safe cosleeping strategies, particularly if you choose to bedshare. Mothers' bodies certainly evolved to sleep next to their infants, but one potential problem is that the recent diverse and complex furniture on which Western mothers and families sleep did not. Other dangerous conditions include when mothers smoke and bedshare, and when an adult in the bed takes drugs or alcohol. How and where your family chooses to cosleep can be adapted, though, or modified, to what you and your baby need in order to sleep as comfortably and as safely as possible.

As explained throughout this book, cosleeping environments require considerable efforts by parents to make them as safe as possible. These efforts can, for parents and infants alike, lead to enormous rewards. It is important to consider the positive impact that the type of cosleeping you choose can have on establishing and maintaining a close bond (especially for parents who are away from the baby many hours during the day), and how it is especially beneficial in supporting the breast-feeding relationship. Now, and throughout history, cosleeping has played an important role in promoting infant survival and well-being, and has always made both short- and long-term contributions to healthy development.

Parents may face opposition from family, child-care experts, and pediatricians, however, who stress the importance of solitary sleep for the child and intimacy for the parents, or who choose to label all bedsharing as unsafe regardless of circumstances. Opponents of cosleeping claim falsely that "problems" are inevitable and that social skills and independence might only be obtained by children through a narrow set of experiences associated with (of all things) solitary sleep experiences that minimize parental interventions and contact. Nothing could be further from the scientific truth.[3] Many well-intentioned people, professional and lay alike, believe that all forms of cosleeping are harmful and cannot be made safe. And yet, to condemn all forms of cosleeping and bedsharing without specifically distinguishing between the safe and unsafe factors, and without considering how benefits and risks vary according to context, is to confuse personal preferences and ideologies with good public policy strategies and better, less biased science.

Hundreds of thousands of babies died from SIDS (the term given to infants who died from unknown causes) in cribs, when used unsafely and without the supervision of an adult caregiver, leading to intensive study into what makes cribs and crib use safe or dangerous. Nobody has ever shown that bedsharing cannot be made safe, only that it can be made unsafe. The presumption made by some medical authorities that a mother is unable to respond to her infant's needs while sleeping is refuted by human infant survival throughout history and prehistory. On a more practical level, such a view is refuted by our own extensive laboratory studies,[4] by cross-cultural data on infancy and bedsharing worldwide[5] and by evolutionary data[6] which has linked mother-infant cosleeping with breastfeeding.

28

Most importantly, the idea that any and all bedsharing is inherently dangerous is refuted by mothers themselves[7] who currently sleep safely with their babies, or did so in the recent past. To perpetuate to the public the idea that the mother's body, no matter what her intentions, motives, and capacities, represents an inherent threat to her infant is not only scientifically unsupportable, but immoral and far more dangerous in the long run, for a variety of reasons, than the idea of cosleeping itself.

I worry more and more about our society's willingness to overlook parental rights, acquired wisdom, and parental judgments in favor of an increasingly impersonal and inappropriate one-size-must-fit-all "medical parenting science." Aside from *getting it wrong* on a scale with which we are already all too tragically familiar (recommendations to place infants on their stomachs to sleep, place infants in separate rooms, and to bottle feed), such a world view, if left unchallenged, further undermines parents' enjoyment of their infants and, worse, leads them to doubt their own abilities to assess what their own infants really need and why, preventing them from making their infants happy, safe and healthy.

SLEEPING WITH YOUR BABY IS NORMAL

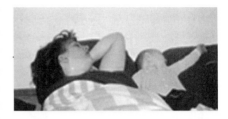

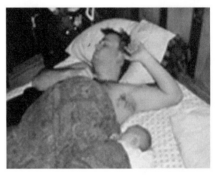

For most of human history (and before written records) covering hundreds of thousands of years, mothers have effectively combined cosleeping and breastfeeding to provide for their babies' immediate social, psychological and physical needs. Human infants are born more helpless than any other animal species. Whether born in Indiana or Papua New Guinea, they are especially vulnerable, slow developing, and must rely on their parents' touch, carrying and feeding for survival. Most mammals are born with 60-90% of adult brain size. Humans are born with just 25% of adult brain size. Compared with other mammals, human infants take the longest time to grow up, and they remain in a biologically dependent state for the longest period of time. In this immature state, human babies are, for the first few months of life at least, unable to efficiently regulate their body temperature without mother being in proximity, and they are unable to make effective antibodies found in mothers' breastmilk to protect themselves from bacteria and viruses. Human infants cannot control their bowels, speak, make tools, digest large molecules, or walk. In the words of anthropologist Ashley Montagu, human infants are "extero-gestators,"[8] meaning they complete their gestation after birth, and someone's got to be there to help with it.

Due to this extreme human developmental immaturity, babies require parental (especially maternal) smell, touch, sounds and movement in order to feel secure and to have their physical needs met at an optimal level. All primate infants, including humans, biologically expect to be in close contact and proximity with their caregivers. In fact, human infants are at birth not adapted to the outside physical environment, but only to what mother's body offers the infant. There is no such thing as giving a human infant too much contact or affection—they thrive on touch, and grow more the more they get of it![9] When deprived of these sensations, a baby will use her primary survival response—crying—and will produce cortisol, a stress hormone, as she attempts to attract the attention of her parents.

Cosleeping, traditionally an extension of our human need for infant-parent closeness, is significant to our evolutionary endurance. Anthropological studies that examined the sleeping customs of families in tropical, non-industrialized cultures have discovered that all of these hunter-gatherer and tribal-level societies share sleep with their babies.[10] Researchers consider these societies to be more similar ecologically and adaptively to prehistoric cultures, whose members coslept in order to ensure their infants' survival and well being. Thus, cosleeping is very, very old among human beings.

It is only in recent history that mothers in a relatively small area of the world have the dubious luxury to ask two basic questions: "How will my baby be fed?" and "Where will my baby sleep?" The advent of these questions stems from the discovery and production of baby formulas, and from society's emphasis on the alleged benefits of bottle feeding. Bottle feeding enabled mothers to spend more time apart from their babies, and with rising affluence in the middle class and an increased value on individualism, separate bedrooms for parents and children became more common and culturally fashionable. By the mid-1900s, it became very common, for the first time in human history, for babies to be bottle fed and then placed to sleep on their stomachs (to promote uninterrupted sleep) in a room far from the sensory range and supervision of their parents. It did not work out very well for babies. Culture changed, but the human infant's need for breastmilk and contact with the mother's body did not.

Along with this trend came another alarming development—babies in increasing numbers were not waking up. Sudden Infant Death Syndrome (SIDS), for which we scientists still have no explanation, grew. We still do not know the exact causes of SIDS, also known as cot or crib death, only that there may well be many causes that interact with a range of possible environmental stressors, not the least of which include maternal smoking, not breastfeeding, and the prone (stomach) infant sleep position. SIDS is diagnosed only following a full toxicological report and post-mortem analysis, when all other causes of death have been ruled out. SIDS remains, then, a "diagnosis by exclusion." When SIDS was first defined as a medical entity in 1963, the death rate from this tragic syndrome was between 2–3 babies per 1000 live baby births in most Western nations. SIDS emerged in Western societies alongside never before tried infant care innovations: artificial milk or cow's milk, prone infant sleep, and infants sleeping alone in rooms by themselves. Coupled with increasingly more mothers smoking before and after their pregnancies, a real SIDS epidemic was in the making.

Researchers now know that placing babies on their stomachs, the prone position, is the most significant risk factor for SIDS, with maternal smoking either before or after the baby's birth coming in at a close second. We see in the data that babies who are fed infant formula die either from SIDS (or from some other congenital abnormality or illness) at higher numbers than babies who are breastfed. And we know that babies who do not share rooms with their parents, but sleep alone in their own room, are sometimes twice as likely to succumb to SIDS, according to recent studies in Great Britain, New Zealand, and a variety of countries in Western Europe.

In many Asian cultures, where cosleeping and breastfeeding (as well as low maternal smoking rates) are the norms, SIDS is either considered rare or is simply unheard of. A baby put to sleep alone in his own room is an image seen only in the last hundred years or so and only in industrialized Western societies. Our culture's emphasis on independence, individualism and self-reliance has helped drive the ideology that babies should sleep alone. Without any developmental evidence supporting such conclusions, it was merely assumed that forced solitariness for infants and children led automatically to secure, independent adults without any sleep problems. These assumptions have hurt us, but it is not too late to return to doing what cultures across the world consider the norm: cosleeping.

COSLEEPING AROUND THE WORLD

For the overwhelming majority of mothers and babies around the globe today, cosleeping is an unquestioned practice. In much of southern Europe, Asia, Africa and Central and South America, mothers and babies routinely share sleep. In many cultures, cosleeping is the norm until chil-

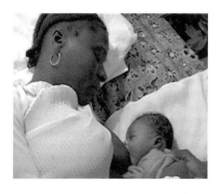

dren are weaned, and some continue long after weaning. Japanese parents (or grandparents) often sleep in proximity with their children until they are teenagers, referring to this arrangement as a river—the mother is one bank, the father another, and the child sleeping between them is the water. Most of the present world cultures practice forms of cosleeping and there are very few cultures in the world for which it would ever even be thought acceptable or desirable to have babies sleeping alone.

Cosleeping is practiced in a variety of ways around the world. In Latin America, the Philippines, and Vietnam, some parents sleep with their baby in a hammock next to the bed. Others place their baby in a wicker basket in the bed, between the two parents. In Japan, many parents sleep next to their baby on bamboo or straw mats, or on futons. Some parents simply roomshare by putting the baby in a crib or bassinet that is kept within arm's reach of the bed. Most cultures that routinely practice cosleeping, in any form, have very rare instances of SIDS. SIDS occurrences are among the lowest in the world in Hong Kong, where cosleeping is extremely common.

Cosleeping is actually more common in the U.S. than most people believe. The typical American home has a room that contains a crib for the baby, and parents report that the baby sleeps in the crib. Yet when researchers ask specific questions about who sleeps where, it turns out that the majority of mothers sleep with their young children at least some of most nights. Parents present themselves as having babies who sleep alone, following the societal norm of the baby in the baby's room and the couple in the master bedroom, but that is not an accurate representation of what is really happening.

The Centers for Disease Control (CDC) in Atlanta collects data that provide information on all means of prenatal and well-baby stressors. Through this, we know that cosleeping is not unusual for American families at all. Roughly 68% of babies enjoyed cosleeping at least some of the time. Further analyses of the data show us that about 26% of infants coslept "always" or "almost always." Combining them with the babies who cosleep "sometimes," it appears that 44% of US babies from 2–9 months old are cosleeping in an adult bed at any given time.[11]

Japan, another industrialized country, not only has one of the lowest infant mortality rates (less than 3 infants per 1000 live births compared with around 7 for the United States), but one of the lowest SIDS rates in the world (between .2 and .3 babies per 1000 live births compared with approximately .5 per 1000 infants for the United States). The Japan SIDS Family Organization reported that SIDS rates continue to decline in Japan as maternal smoking approaches practically 0, and exclusive breastfeeding reaches around 70–75%. In fact, one report shows that as bedsharing and breastfeeding increased and as maternal smoking decreased, SIDS rates decreased. This suggests yet again that it is not necessarily bedsharing, but how it is practiced, that can be dangerous.

Interestingly, it may be that Japanese bedsharing rates do not differ all that much from those in the United States, but the cultural acceptance of cosleeping as the norm is very different. In 1998, 60% of parents said they practiced bedsharing in Japan, only about 16% more than US parents. This means that the practice of cosleeping does not necessarily vary a great deal from culture to culture, but rather that the social acceptance of cosleeping is what varies.

HOW THE ANIMALS DO IT

"For species such as primates, the mother is the environment."
SARAH BLAFFER HRDY, 1999

Mammals instinctually remain close to their young. Their babies would not survive without the warmth, food, protection and psychological nourishment their mothers provide. All mammals cosleep in one form or another; when and how this takes place, however, varies according to the mother's overall ecological adaptations, including her relationship to the male of the species, and her own nutritional and maintenance requirements.

Some mothers (such as migrating whales and polar bears) fast while the babies are young, using their stores of body fat to sustain themselves and produce breastmilk. Others (like the big cats) share the tasks of child-minding and hunting so that the community ensures that both tasks get done. A significant number of mammal mothers leave their young hidden away (beneath low-lying shrubs, up in trees, or in dens, burrows, caves or lairs) while they forage for the food they need to sustain themselves and to make milk for their babies. These mammals are called the "nested species." The babies of these nested species do not cry when their mothers leave in part because if they did predators

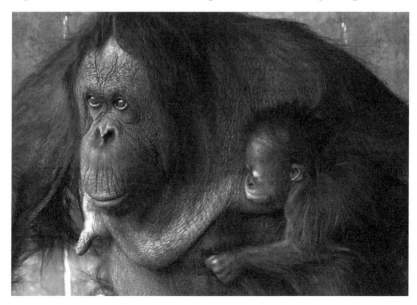

would be able to hear and track them, but mostly because their mothers' milk is so rich in fat that, after nursing, they remain satisfied during their mothers' absence. For example, fawns are hidden in nests beneath bushes and remain alone for periods as long as 8–10 hours. Deer milk is 19 % fat, allowing these babies to stay full until their mother returns. Then, the babies will nurse again and the entire family, including the mother and siblings, will sleep nestled together.

Unlike these nested species, primate mammals, such as monkeys, apes and humans, are referred to by scientists as the "carrying species." Our milk contains more water and sugar and about 10 %–20 % less fat than that of the nested species. Fat is the growth nutrient and mammals with low fat content in their breastmilk grow at a slower rate than those animals who drink fat-rich milk. After nursing, primate mammals are only satisfied for 1–2 hours before they are ready to eat again to eliminate their hunger. This need to breastfeed frequently means that primate mammals, in contrast to babies of the nesting species, must stay close to their mothers. Hence, rather than being safely tucked away somewhere, primate infants are carried until they reach at least 6–12 months of age and usually until they are much older. Primate babies will sleep in their mother's arms or while clinging to their backs so that the infant becomes integrated into almost every aspect of the mother's daily routine.

This constant physical contact ensures that a physiological as well as a social bond is established between mother and baby, one that enables the neurologically immature primate newborn to develop and function more efficiently. Physical contact compensates for the fact that human newborns cannot shiver to keep themselves warm and are unable to make sufficient antibodies that come in mothers' milk. The sensation of touch itself stimulates the release of endorphins that help the baby's immature gut absorb the calories needed for growth. Developmental psychologist Dr. Tiffany Field found that human babies who were massaged fifteen minutes per day experienced a remarkable 47 % increase in daily weight gain compared with those infants who were not massaged.[12]

For us carrying species, then, the parents have an especially significant role in making growth possible! When an infant monkey is separated from its mother, it is hard for the baby—it experiences a loss of body temperature, an irregular heart rhythm, higher stress levels, and will, in extreme cases, become so clinically depressed that it eventually dies. Human infants, who are the least neurologically mature primates and are fed with breastmilk that is especially low in fat, depend on adult contact. Remember, human babies have been likened by anthropologist Ashley Montagu to little kangaroo joeys which develop fully insulated within their mothers' pouches. Montagu stresses that our puny 25 % brain volume at birth relative to our adult size explains why we are unable to cling to our mother's chests for easy transportation the way monkey and ape babies do.[13] Basically we are all born "preemies" compared with other mammalian species. Like the kangaroo joey, the human infant's central nervous system depends on having a micro-environment that is similar to the maternal uterine environment from which it came, an environment full of sensory exchanges involving heat, sound, movement, transportation, feelings, touch, smells, and of course access to nutrients from mother's breast. As infants, human beings are not biologically designed nor prepared to be separated from their mothers. Separation can be tantamount to a death sentence.

COSLEEPING IS GOOD FOR BABIES

baby who sleeps in proximity to her parents is reassured by the continual reminders of the caregivers' presence—touches, smell, movement, warmth and, by virtue of increased breastfeeding, taste. These sensations provide emotional security for the baby, and, if the newborn is breastfeeding, a steady supply of signals and cues (such as fragrances from mother's milk) promotes more breastfeeding and increased nourishment. If your baby's well-being is threat-

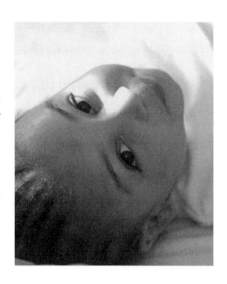

ened—for example, if he is choking or struggling to move a blanket away from his face—you will (if attentive) be able to help right away. In such a protected and nurturing environment, your baby will benefit from an almost immediate response to his or her needs.

When babies, especially before they can verbalize their needs, do not have their needs met, they cry. Crying evolved as an alarm signal reserved for critical circumstances involving pain, hunger or fear, and it is used to elicit mothers' retrieval behavior. Years ago it was learned that prolonged crying decreases oxygenation and increases heart rate which in turn then augments cortisol, a stress hormone previously discussed.

Some studies have suggested that elevated levels of cortisol in infancy can cause physical changes in the brain, prompting a greater vulnerability to social attachment disorders. At the very least, the energy lost in crying could be better put into growth or maintenance.[14] Babies who cosleep are much less likely to cry themselves to sleep, or even cry at all, and so avoid releasing an excess of this hormone. However, many parents are now encouraged to use "controlled crying techniques" to manage infants and young children who do not settle alone, who wake at night, or who settle only if held or permitted to sleep in proximity or contact with the parents. So concerned is the Australian Association of Infant Mental Health about the use of such techniques that they issued the following statement: "…controlled crying is not consistent with what infants need for their optimal emotional and psychological health, and may have unintended negative consequences."[15]

Babies are warmer when they sleep next to their moms, reducing the need for heavy or numerous blankets. Throughout the night mothers and infants are exchanging sensory experiences, such as body heat, that serve to regulate the baby's state. When a newly-born infant is removed from his mother's uterus, for example, the baby can experience a loss of up to one degree Fahrenheit of body temperature, generally explained yet again by the production of stress hormones. This drop in temperature can reduce immunity, making a baby more susceptible to infectious diseases, and takes energy away from growth and development in an attempt to regulate the baby's temperature. One study found that among 11- to 16-week-old infants, babies that slept alone had a lower average axillary (underarm) skin temperature than babies who breastfed and slept alongside their mothers.[16]

Babies that sleep with their mothers and breastfeed spend less time in the deepest stages of sleep (stage three and stage four), from which arousal is more difficult should the baby need to awaken quickly to terminate a dangerous apnea (episodes in which one stops breathing). Instead, cosleeping babies spend more time in lighter stages of sleep (stage one and stage two). Light stage sleep is thought to be physiologically more appropriate for young infants, and more natural and conducive to safe sleep for babies, because it is easier to awaken to terminate apneas than it is when babies are in deeper stages of sleep. The shorter durations of deeper stage sleep promoted by cosleeping can potentially protect those infants born with arousal deficiencies (suspected to be involved in SIDS). Moreover, cosleeping significantly increases the total nightly number of infant arousals as the baby gets a lot of practice in arousing to mother's external sounds, movements and touches. This increase in arousals may improve her ability to develop awakening skills that can prove handy should the infant's oxygen supply decrease following a breathing pause. The baby not only stirs in relationship to mother's movements, but the smells of mother's breastmilk nearby also contribute to the infant's tendency to remain in light sleep for a longer period of time.[17]

Ironically, increased arousals with oxygenations and remaining for longer periods of time in lighter stages of sleep (all natural consequences of breastfeeding with cosleeping), are the same consequences associated with pacifier use. Those opposed to bedsharing who served on the American Academy of Pediatrics panel argued that mothers should use pacifiers as one possible way to prevent SIDS as a result of the consequences listed above! Wouldn't it be nice if these same researchers had as much faith in what mother's own body can contribute as they do in these fake nipples?

Both pre- and full-term infants can benefit significantly from the physical presence of their parents, although as I mention later, I do not recommend that premature infants actually sleep in the bed with their mothers due to their increased vulnerability and small size. Nonetheless, aside from the ability of infants to learn at a faster rate due to the greater number of social interactions and frequent communicative patterns that come with increased contact and proximity, scientific studies show that when babies rest on their mothers' or fathers' chests, enjoying direct skin-to-skin contact, they breathe more regularly, use energy more efficiently, grow faster, and experience less stress.[18] In several recent reviews, Dr. Sari Goldstein, Dr. Makhuaul and Dr. Helen Ball point out that skin-to-skin contact, sometimes referred to as kangaroo care, leads to earlier discharge of premature infants, fewer apneas and fewer bradycardia incidents (periods of slow heart rates).[19] Maternal contact is known to act as a pain killer for newborns and increased touching and holding helps infants to recover rapidly from birth-related fatigue.[20] Spontaneous breastfeeding is also facilitated by contact as well as serving to encourage the mother to continue to breastfeed for longer periods of time per breastfeeding session.[21] Sleep duration is increased among infants who experience skin-to-skin care, and they seem less agitated in general while enjoying more stable heart rate and breathing patterns leading to greater overall oxygenation.[22]

There are also benefits for mothers. Skin-to-skin contact is associated with a significant increase in maternal oxytocin levels (a hormone released during breastfeeding) in two Swedish studies,[23] which suggests that uterine contraction would be enhanced and milk ejection improved, to the benefit of both mother and infant. Finally, there is a report that skin-to-skin contact is also associated with lowered maternal anxiety and more efficient participation of mothers in caring for their newborn infants.[24]

Letting a baby cry herself to sleep is advice given to parents with the goal of raising a child that is self-reliant, able to comfort herself and comfortable with aloneness. Researchers are now finding that in extreme cases leaving children to cry without offering any comfort can cause lasting damage to their brains. Persistent distress as a child is being linked with higher rates of depression and emotional problems later in life. Many child psychologists now believe that babies know best, and parents should follow the instinct that directs them to try to soothe a crying baby.

As a developmental extension of the skin-to-skin experience, parent-infant bedsharing, when practiced safely, can be a warm and snuggly experience that many parents enjoy. However, it is much more than that—it is a biologically-driven process whereby the baby's body temperature is regulated and steady breathing is promoted in part by the sounds of mother's breathing and by the infant feeling the mother's rhythmic chest movements. In many biological studies these cues are shown to act as "hidden" stimuli by which the young of other mammals time their next breath![25,26]

Even the mother's expelled carbon dioxide (CO_2) is not wasted in a cosleeping situation; the amount of CO_2 the mother expires in her breath acts to stimulate infant breathing.[27] Expelled CO_2 appears to act as a potential back-up should the baby's own internal drive to breathe falters or slows, since the baby's nasal regions can both detect and respond to the presence of this gas by breathing faster.

And there are still more advantages to parent-infant contact. During skin-to-skin contact, the infant body stimulates just the right brain cells to be nurtured and connected to each other. In a sense, nighttime cosleeping can be said to extend the needed micro-environment that during the day also fosters a variety of social, communicative, and emotional skills while the baby is being monitored and protected. A mother is certainly more than a service provider; she is the entity around which the human infant was designed not just to be awake, but to sleep. The English psychologist Donald Winnicott spoke of the baby's profound dependence on others for life-sustaining support when he said, "There is no such thing as a baby, there is a baby and someone." When considering what infants need or trying to explain what infants can or cannot do, **nothing** makes sense except in relation to the mother's body.

WHY COSLEEPING IS IMPORTANT TO BREASTFEEDING

For breastfeeding mothers, cosleeping can ease interruptions caused by nighttime feedings. The American Academy of Pediatrics Section on Breastfeeding recommends that mothers and infants should sleep in proximity to each other to facilitate breastfeeding,[28] and while the Task Force on Infant Sleep and SIDS calls bedsharing "hazardous," they too recommend roomsharing. For the first time in American history, all pediatric scientists agree that cosleeping in the form of roomsharing should be supported, not only because it

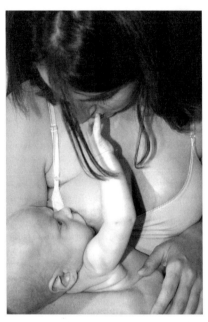

facilitates breastfeeding, but because a mother sleeping proximate to her infant reduces the infant's chances of SIDS, as recent evidence reveals.[29] Aside from this, several studies show that breastfeeding mothers and newborns get more rest when they cosleep.[30] It's much easier to breastfeed bedside than to get up and walk down the hall to another room and then try to resettle a baby who wants only to be touched by his mother.

Mothers who bedshare often report they hardly need to awaken when the baby is hungry or that they need only awaken for a few minutes to get the baby latched on. The baby nurses as needed and Mom continues to sleep, yet with an awareness of how the baby is doing. Babies should not have to cry in order to be fed, according to the American Academy of Pediatrics Section on Breastfeeding and other lactation scientists, who agree that "crying is a late indicator of hunger."[31] Of course the best way, perhaps the only way, to know if your baby is hungry without the baby crying is to be close enough to hear the baby's sounds and to feel the baby's wiggles and arm movements, which act as nonverbal invitations to feed.

Recall that the composition of human milk creates a short hunger cycle in human babies, who need to feed often. Anthropologist Carol Worthman from Emory University followed breastfeeding Kalahari !Kung Bushman mothers and babies around all day as mothers gathered their nuts and berries. She found that throughout the day these carried babies snacked on breastmilk every 13 minutes for a few minutes at a time! By keeping babies close, or by using breast pumps in Western societies, mothers can more easily meet their babies' nutritional needs. In fact, nighttime research shows that the average breastfeeding interval of routinely bedsharing mothers is close to an hour and a half, or the length of the human sleep cycle.[32] This raises the possibility that the nutritional needs of cosleeping and breastfeeding infants has determined the average length of an adult sleep cycle, and supports the idea that appropriate cosleeping practices, especially when combined with nighttime breastfeeding, is innate and clinically beneficial human behavior.

Our own intensive laboratory studies in which mothers and infants are filmed through infrared cameras reveal that babies who are breastfed and share a bed with their mothers tend to nurse more often than breastfeeding mothers and infants sleeping in separate rooms, and for longer periods.[33] One large scale study comparing breast, mixed and bottle feeding infants' weight gain showed that, among the breastfed infants, higher weight gain was associated with more frequent feeding.[34]

Frequent breastfeeding ensures also that infants receive greater immunological benefits. The more often babies nurse and the more breastmilk they are given, the more antibodies they receive—designer antibodies, too, produced in kind by the mother specifically to fight bacteria found in the infant's own home environment, and any viruses or bacteria to which the mother and baby are exposed. For newborns, who are particularly vulnerable to disease because of their immature immune systems, these antibodies can provide vital protection from dangerous and potentially fast-acting fatal infectious diseases.[35]

While our studies here in the United States have demonstrated how bedsharing promotes a significantly higher number of nightly breastfeeds among bedsharing mothers compared with breastfeeding mothers and infants with separate sleep spaces, Dr. Ball's studies in Durham, Great Britain show how the greater convenience of bedsharing tends to promote a greater commitment by breastfeeding mothers to breastfeed for a greater number of months, contributing health benefits to infants and mothers alike.[36]

Until relatively recently we had no scientific evidence regarding how many infant lives breastfeeding might save in industrialized nations. But even in a country such as the United States, where infectious diseases are mostly under control due to our strict sanitary practices, a recent epidemiological study showed that approximately 720 American babies die each year from congenital or infectious diseases, or illness complications, because they were not breastfed.[37] This was the first study to show that even in a highly industrialized Western culture, such as in the United States, breastfeeding saves infants' lives.

As well as benefiting the health of your baby, breastfeeding also provides emotional and cognitive benefits, including the opportunity to learn and practice communicative cues as newborns. Your baby will let you know when it's time to nurse, and will be gratified by your immediate response. Maybe this is why breastfed babies score higher on IQ tests and other cognitive tests: not only is breastmilk the primary and best architect of the infant's brain, but babies are generally happier and more willing to engage with their environments.[38]

Epidemiological, laboratory and observational studies also reveal that while babies certainly benefit from mothers breastfeeding them, in turn, the infants' sucking, especially when it is often and prolonged over a great number of months, contributes to mothers' short- and long-term health. For example, breastfeeding helps return the mother's uterus to its prepregnant size, works to help the mother retain iron, and delays the return of ovulation which increases the birth interval. The shorter the intervals between feeds, the more powerful this contraceptive effect and the better for the mother overall. Most importantly, breastfeeding helps to protect mothers from various kinds of reproductive cancers, especially breast cancer. The World Health Organization, for example, sponsored a study of 5,878 cases of breast cancer comparing them with 8,216 controls (women who did not get cancer) and found that as the number of lifetime months of breastfeeding increased, a woman's chances of getting breast cancer were diminished, especially if she breastfed for between 15–40 months of her life. If she did so she had only a 30–40 % chance of getting breast cancer compared with women who never breastfed, or who did so for only a few months.[39]

Another rather remarkable study describes a fishing village in Hong Kong in which breastfeeding mothers do something we might think odd: the women in this village breastfeed their infants from only one breast! This amounts to the ultimate controlled experiment since both breasts were exposed to the identical environmental factors and physiological experiences with only one exception: one breast was used for suckling and the other was not. Guess which breast did not become cancerous? Yes! The suckled breast seemed to be protected.[40]

BENEFITS OF COSLEEPING FOR THE BREASTFED BABY
(WHEN KNOWN ADVERSE FACTORS ARE ABSENT)

- Greater breastmilk supply
  As babies breastfeed throughout the night, their suckling stimulates their mothers to create more of the milk needed for proper nourishment.

- More frequent breastfeeding
  Studies tell us that more frequent infant feeds reduce crying duration, thereby contributing to your baby's energy conservation and calm wakefulness.

- Longer breastfeeding sessions
  Longer feeds ensure that your baby receives enough daily calories to provide adequate nutrition and weight gain.

- Longer breastfeeding period
  By continually breastfeeding over time, babies receive the immunological and nutritional benefits they need for optimum growth and development.

- Increased safety
  Breastfeeding babies are being constantly monitored throughout the night, and tend to be placed on their backs, in the recommended supine position, with their noses and mouths unobstructed.

- Increased infant sleep duration
  Babies who sleep alone must cry loudly enough to wake their parents who are sleeping several rooms away. By sleeping together, babies achieve a longer and better rest period.

- Lower stress levels
  When babies do not have to cry to have their needs met, thus becoming agitated, they are able to stay calmer and more content.

- Temperature regulation
  Babies are warmer when they sleep next to their moms, and mothers can sense their baby's temperature and respond by adding a blanket if her infant seems chilled or by removing covers if her infant is overheated.

- Increased sensitivity to mother's communication
  Moms and babies who routinely sleep together have a heightened and enhanced sensitivity to each other's smells, movements and touches.

BENEFITS OF COSLEEPING FOR THE BREASTFEEDING MOTHER (WHEN KNOWN ADVERSE FACTORS ARE ABSENT)

- Greater breastmilk supply
  Breastfeeding on demand throughout the night helps mothers establish and maintain their milk supply.

- Increased protection from breast and other reproductive cancers
  Bedsharing increases both breastfeeding frequency and duration in months, increasing the cancer-protective effects of long-term breastfeeding.

- More rapid excess weight loss after pregnancy

- Enhanced attachment and parental fulfillment
  Especially for working mothers, increased time with baby during the night enhances attachment and helps the mother to feel fulfilled as a parent.

- Reassurance that baby is safe
  Most breastfeeding mothers who routinely bedshare with their babies tend to place their babies on their backs, and sleep in a position that keeps the baby from burrowing under pillows or quilts.

- Increased sleep duration for mother
  Studies have demonstrated that mothers who sleep with their babies have more sleep and evaluate their sleep more positively than do mothers that sleep apart from their infants.

- Lower stress levels
  The increased nipple contact that occurs during nocturnal breastfeeds works to increase the mother's production of oxytocin, a hormone that contributes to a sense of calm and well-being.

- Increased sensitivity to baby's communication
  Mothers are able to respond quickly if an infant wants to feed, thus lowering anxiety that the baby's needs are not being met.

WHY COSLEEPING IS IMPORTANT TO THOSE WHO FORMULA FEED

Although breastfeeding is best, not all mothers choose to or are able to breastfeed. Regardless of feeding method, however, all human infants benefit emotionally and psychologically by sensing, knowing and reacting to their parents' contact and proximity, and the parents also 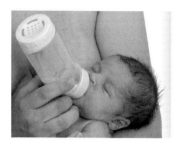 benefit by being close to their infants. A number of studies show that attachment and maternal sensitivity, as well as emotional bonding, is improved through increased physical holding and carrying. This increased contact acts to reduce the chances of future child abuse and neglect among high risk mothers and babies, especially socio-economically deprived mother-baby pairs.[41, 42, 43]

That being said, one reason why I am generally more concerned about the safety of bedsharing for bottle feeding mother-baby pairs is because those of us that have studied breast vs. bottle feeding mother-baby sleep patterns have noticed that breastfeeding mothers and babies, more so than bottle feeding mothers and babies, tend to sleep facing each other, and breastfeeding mothers tend to tuck their knees up underneath their babies, often sleeping on their sides, which seems to be related to both the positioning for breastfeeding and the communication patterns that unfold in a bedsharing and breastfeeding context. In Great Britain, Dr. Helen Ball, who runs the University of Durham Parent Sleep Center (www.dur.ac.uk/sleep.lab), studied differences between bottle feeding and breastfeeding dyads and noted that breastfeeding and bedsharing mothers and babies tend to arouse more quickly in response to the other's stirrings than do bottle feeding and bedsharing mothers and babies, suggesting greater conditioned mutual sensitivity that can enhance safety.[44] Perhaps, then, while skin-to-skin contact could occur during periods in which the infant is awake during the night, it is probably best for most families who bottle feed to cosleep by placing the infant next to the bed on a different surface rather than to sleep with the baby in the bed, although, as always, you are in the best position to judge exactly how sensitive and responsive you can be to your baby. A mother's motivation and intent matter here. But, as always, it is important not to bedshare if the right conditions cannot be maintained.

The good news is that if the safety of nighttime bedsharing cannot be maintained (if, for example, you have too small a bed, or other older children crawl in unexpectedly) there are other ways to facilitate safe body contact between mothers and infants that can also enhance attachment and thus increase the infant's and the mother's health and happiness. For example, among low income mothers, Anisfeld's research team explored the effects of increased physical contact as achieved through the regular use of a soft infant carrier on the mother-infant relationship. They found that this "experimental intervention," providing mothers with infant carriers, significantly increased the mother's responsiveness to her infant's vocalizations when the child was three and a half months old, and further promoted the establishment of a secure attachment at 13 months. This research showed that this extended closeness may have made it possible for more stressed mothers to learn how to properly respond to their babies' needs and to enjoy their infants more while doing so.[45]

Surely, both breast and bottle feeding babies respond positively to hearing mother's movements, touches, and breathing, and they are reassured and physiologically affected by mother's presence. The more mother and infant are in close proximity, the better each gets at interpreting and responding in kind to each other's signals and cues, and communication is enhanced. This is especially important to bottle fed babies who might miss out on some of the intense bonding that takes place during breastfeeding. The bottle fed baby definitely sleeps more safely when Mom and Dad are close by (though in different beds) since proximity permits an attentive parent to respond to dangerous situations, such as Baby getting her head covered or rolling over on her stomach. Mom and Dad can always come to the rescue when they are near.

BENEFITS OF SEPARATE SURFACE COSLEEPING FOR THE FORMULA-FED BABY AND PARENTS

- Nurturing sleep environment.
  Cosleeping babies are more confident that their needs will be met almost immediately, and mothers and fathers who sleep close by their babies are able to respond quickly if their infant cries, chokes, needs his nasal passages cleared, needs to be cooled or warmed, or simply to be held.

- Emotionally reassuring
  Babies who sleep with their parents receive the comfort of their mothers' and fathers' touch, warmth and protection. For parents who work outside the home, separate surface cosleeping can be a wonderfully restorative time to reconnect with their baby.

- Safety
  Depending on the degree of the mother's desire to sleep in contact with her infant, and her capacity or ability to sustain a safe bedsharing environment, side-by-side cosleeping (on different surfaces) and roomsharing (rather than bedsharing) may well be the safest and most reassuring way to cosleep for the bottle fed mother-infant pair.

- Lower stress
  Your presence can be extremely reassuring if your baby is ill or irritable, and your ability to immediately monitor your baby's state can provide peace of mind throughout the night.

- More sleep
  Separate surface cosleeping babies cry less frequently and sleep more often, and if you are right next to your baby, you can meet his needs without having to get out of bed and retrieve him from his crib.

How Parents Can Benefit From Cosleeping

here are now several different studies[46, 47, 48] focusing on why parents choose to cosleep in the form of bedsharing, and it appears there exist myriad reasons for doing so, and the most prominent reason among the many found is that "everyone gets more sleep." This response is related to the other primary reasons: because mothers find it much easier to breastfeed if bedsharing, and it "just feels right." A cross-cultural survey of over 200 families from the USA, Great Britain, France, Canada, Australia and New Zealand revealed that fears of not getting to babies fast enough during an earthquake or fire, of SIDS or of the sudden onset of a serious illness or fever, and even concerns about the baby being lonely all appeared in the picture of why families cosleep. "Peaceful," "comforting," "loving" and "protective" are words that showed up repeatedly in parental descriptions of what bedsharing means to them. "I work in an office all day long; cosleeping is a way to reconnect," said one mother.

Then there are some reasons for bedsharing that one might not think of, such as when some infants, or parents, may be blind or deaf. One mother, sightless from birth, wrote: "How could I have ever mothered my darling baby without having him nestled up right near me? It gave

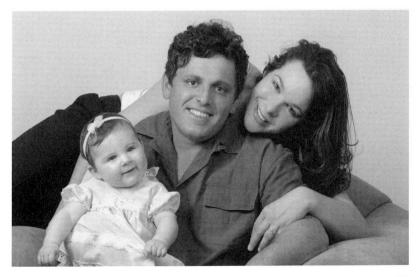

me total fulfillment as a parent and my son could have cared less that I was sightless and, indeed, because of his utmost joy of me being close to him, I would often forget that I was, in fact, blind." And the mother of a deaf and blind baby contributed: "I always felt a little weird about (my son) being in the dark and unable to hear, so once I gave up my 'preconceived notions' that children sleeping in their parents' bed was bad, bedtime has been much more peaceful."[49]

One mother of two deaf infants participated in our study. She wrote: "I have two deaf boys, now 5 and 8. They both slept with us until this last year. We began by accident (to bedshare) when nursing them made it much easier. When we found out the oldest was deaf we were so happy we had made that decision. Because they could not hear at night...they felt much more comfortable with us near them." And finally one mother writes: "My mother's parents were deaf-mutes and the doctor insisted they sleep with their children. She [my grandmother] laid the babies at the head of the bed on a pillow and slept with her hand on the baby all night."

Some families cannot afford cribs, so for these mothers there is no choice but to sleep on the same surface with their infants. Seeing the baby whenever you wake, watching the baby's chest rise up and down with each breath, hearing the baby (even if just a sigh or a faint sound), covering him if he's kicked off the blanket, wrapping your finger in his—these are the actions that sustain new parents and help them cherish the little life before them.

Peace of mind is significant, but the benefits for Mom and Dad don't stop there (when bedsharing is chosen by the parent and done safely, of course). Helen Ball's study of cosleeping fathers in England, the only study of its kind, found that the dads in her sample were initially reluctant to bedshare, yet they ended up finding the experience overall "more enjoyable than disruptive." She suggests that the intimate contact that dads can have with babies in bed with them helps them to develop, when they want to do so, an intense social relationship with their infants that might otherwise be delayed during breastfeeding. Dr. Ball suggests that "Triadic cosleeping arrangements may serve to ameliorate this effect, and provide fathers who are motivated to do so the opportunity to experience intimate contact and prolonged close interaction with their newborn baby."[50]

WHY DO PEOPLE SAY IT'S DANGEROUS?

"Talk about double standards—while every catastrophic bedsharing death represents to some medical authorities a valid reason to indict and to make an argument against all bedsharing, each and every one of the thousands upon thousands of crib SIDS deaths represents a 'tragic problem to be solved' rather than a 'practice to eliminate.'"

JAMES J. MCKENNA, National Public Radio interview (September 2005)

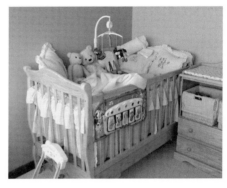

Where babies sleep has emerged as a controversial issue in the medical community. In Western industrialized societies, cosleeping has never been discussed on what anyone could even remotely consider a level playing field. Ideas about the "necessity" of having your baby sleep alone happened to begin around the same time as the emphasis on the supposed superiority of bottle feeding to breastfeeding. These ideas became one and the same with standard medicine, and many decades later medicine emerged to systematically study only bottle fed babies who slept by themselves, characteristic only of infants sleeping in Western industrialized societies. These are the long-standing biases embedded within the medical community, helping those behind the negative headlines to build a case against cosleeping without being asked to reveal all of the relevant facts about infant deaths that are required to truly understand them.[51]

Early 20th-century medical models of "normal, healthy infant sleep" emphasized the importance of minimizing nighttime touch between parents and their infants and children. Ideas quickly developed that solitary sleep would promote the relationship between the parents and help a child to become independent, along with the idea that any form of cosleeping was psychologically damaging or dangerous and denied children the opportunity to grow into competent individuals. Guidelines about why infants should sleep alone seemed more to do with creating good moral character (defined as being a self-sufficient adult) than they seemed designed to help create a physically or psychologically healthy child. Infants sleeping in any form with their parents was discouraged, ignored altogether as a possibility, or described as being perverse or weird.[52]

If we can assume that baby boomers' moms listened to the renowned and respected Dr. Spock, a pediatrician who wrote the canonical parenting guide of the 1950s, then we can see the irony of Dr. Spock's advice for solitary infant sleep: supposedly it would produce adults with "good sleep practices and hygiene," but instead it produced one of the most sleep-deprived adult populations known. Although so many of us were taught to sleep alone as infants on the basis of this advice, more American adults are now sleeping less than six hours a night (the average is a mere 6.8 hours), and 75% of us have difficulty either falling asleep or staying asleep—and all of this is especially true for women! If there is a relationship between early solitary infant sleep experiences and adult sleep, it hardly looks like a good one, and seems to be the opposite of what was promised would actually happen.[53]

> *"Perhaps the American veneration of unbroken sleep is another culturally determined prejudice, posing as science."*
> JOHN SEABROOK, *The New Yorker* (October 1999)

History is not only a possible explanation as to why Westerners sleep so poorly, but also a reason why in the public arena, bedsharing or cosleeping (often incorrectly used interchangeably) is so easily made to look so dangerous, and why people are so willing to be convinced that bedsharing is inherently deadly without knowing the details of how infants who bedshared actually died. One reason why bedsharing comes out looking so dangerous in public news accounts is that when deaths of babies in beds are reported in the media, they are rarely given any context. No details such as whether the parent was drinking beforehand, whether or not the infant's mother smoked during her pregnancy, or whether or not other children were in the bed sleeping next to the infant are ever mentioned. It is as if these factors do not matter, when in fact they likely explain how and why the baby died. Other important factors pertinent to explaining each death are generally omitted in favor of sensationalistic characterizations, like claiming that "cosleeping has killed yet another baby," while the details remain hidden or are simply regarded as less important than the act of bedsharing itself.

Frequently, forms of cosleeping are presented to parents in terms of the "inevitable problems" that might arise if it were practiced. Unlike problems associated with getting babies to sleep alone, and unlike efforts made toward solving the safety issues of babies sleeping in cribs, any possible problems associated with cosleeping are deemed not worth solving, or impossible to solve. **These are social judgments, not science.** In magazine articles and books that take a negative stance on various forms of cosleeping, each infant death is usually used as "proof" of the dangers of bedsharing, and the whole practice is condemned. But each one of the thousands of infants that have died in cribs is NOT used as proof that crib sleeping needs to be eliminated. Because the true causes of almost all bedsharing deaths reported publicly are omitted, it is easy to understand how many of our citizens fail to realize that this "proof" is actually just a bias that the writer of the article or book has, and that it is not proper scientific proof that bedsharing is invariably dangerous and cannot be made safe.

Another reason why so many Westerners criticize cosleeping is that for decades, and without any data at all, psychologists (who now largely support cosleeping) warned families that cosleeping leads to marital discord or divorce—an idea that has since been completely refuted. It was also believed that cosleeping led to sibling jealousies, which, while possible, is most likely only one of many causes of sibling jealousy! Without considering whether the particular parents involved consider cosleeping a bad habit or a good habit, or how cosleeping fits into a family's values, parents are warned that cosleeping creates a "bad habit which is difficult to break." Furthermore, cosleeping is said to confuse the infant or child emotionally or sexually, or to induce over-stimulation. Yet no evidence is ever offered as to how, when, and under what circumstances this could be true and mostly such views have been refuted by studies published in the last fifteen years or so. Even Richard Ferber, the guru of solitary infant sleep, has expressed regrets about his own statements that cosleeping reflected maternal pathologies or caused "confusion or anxiety" among infants, much to his credit.[54]

Unfortunately, many Western medical groups adopted what in my opinion and others' is a wrong solution to the bedsharing controversy. Many medical authorities choose not to disclose the details of bedshar-

> "Our government's recent warning that it was unsafe to ever have babies or small children in bed with parents went way too far... It should be challenged because it's bad science. Bad science sets out to make a point, looks neither to the left nor to the right, but only straight ahead for evidence that supports the point it sets out to make. When it finds evidence it likes, it gathers it tenderly and subjects it to little or no testing."
>
> K. Vonnegut, *The Boston Globe* (October 24, 1999)

ing deaths, but believe instead that the public needs "one simple negative message—never do it."[55] But such a simple message misrepresents the nature and quality of the mother-infant relationship by overly simplifying a complex and highly variable phenomenon. Simple negative messages ignore valid alternative public and professional positions including sound scientific data and perspectives refuting the validity and accuracy of such "simple" messages. These policies underestimate parents' ability to make their own decisions and to make a safe cosleeping environment for their infant, and deny them the opportunity to become fully informed, making it impossible to decide what is best for their family. These are decisions that belong **only** to parents, and not to outside "authorities."[56]

Being able to feel comfortable and well-informed about your choice to bedshare, then, requires a little extra education and possibly some new ways of thinking about ideas that emerge from isolated tragic examples of unsafe bedsharing, or from weak and faulty epidemiological studies. It is very helpful to learn how to respond to negative newspaper or evening news reports, public condemnations of bedsharing by medical authorities, county coroners or infant fatality review board members, or disheartening comments from other parents.

Critical additional factors that need to be included by public officials when reporting infant deaths while bedsharing are such things as whether or not the dead infant was sleeping prone (on her stomach) while bedsharing, if any children were in the bed sleeping next to the baby, whether or not the mother smoked during her pregnancy, whether or not the mother knew how to eliminate gaps or spaces between her mattress and furniture or the bed frame, or whether or not the baby was exclusively breastfed or breastfed at all. These are some examples of independent risk factors for SIDS, and they are what you need to consider when reading about deaths "caused by bedsharing" because they are most likely the real reasons that bedsharing babies die. Public "warnings" about cosleeping ordinarily use the term cosleeping indiscriminately as a catch-all category to include babies dying on couches, sofas, recliners, or armchairs—as if those forms of cosleeping (known to be dangerous) are no more dangerous or carry the same risk factor as safe bedsharing involving a non-smoking, breastfeeding mother.

No scientist who has ever actually studied bedsharing, either in the home or laboratory, or who has studied the physiology and associated behavior involved in bedsharing, has ever recommended against it. In the scientific world, only researchers who study outcomes from extremely large epidemiological studies that fail to appreciate the importance of individual family differences recommend against bedsharing. These scientists do not have any first hand experience studying the very phenomenon they claim to understand. This is not what "evidence-based medicine" is supposed to be about. Patient values, motivations, scientific consensus and respect for variability are equally as important to the formulation of public health recommendations, and not simply population statistics derived from large epidemiological studies.

> "'I was just trying to be a loving mother': Baby's death in parents' bed stirs debate on safe sleep practices—experts divided."
>
> Tim Evans, *Indy Star* (February 7, 2006)

When a baby dies in a crib, attention is given to the specifics of how the baby died, such as whether or not the baby was sleeping prone (on her stomach) or supine (on her back—the safe position). If the baby slept prone in the crib, very likely it will be said that the baby died from SIDS due to sleeping prone; however, if that same baby had died while sleeping prone in an adult bed, the cause of death would likely be said to be from having bedshared, rather than from SIDS due to having slept prone. The preliminary judgment will likely be that the baby suffocated, or that cause of death simply cannot be determined.

In the bedsharing scenario there is a very good chance that SIDS will be excluded as the cause of death by virtue of the fact that the baby died while bedsharing, even without knowledge of how the bedsharing was practiced. Asphyxiation, and not SIDS, will be assumed. In my own state of Indiana, bedsharing babies are assumed to have been suffocated if they are found to have died while bedsharing, and the same is true in Ohio (as was carefully explained to me by a colleague working in the state medical examiner's office). In many areas across the country an ideologically-based diagnostic shift is taking place. The ideology claiming that bedsharing is always deadly is unfortunately taking precedence over careful post-mortem and death scene studies. Ideologically-based judgments provide further statistical evidence for negative assumptions about how bedsharing works.

The fear of suffocating an infant while sleeping is real, but has been grossly exaggerated. Data from the Sudden Unexpected Deaths in Infancy study, the largest such study yet conducted, found that for infants who shared a room with a parent, the risk of SIDS was approximately half that of infants who slept alone. *In other words, putting a baby to sleep in a separate room (rather than the room in which the parents slept) doubled the risk of SIDS.*[57] In reporting a careful description of how 60 Australian babies died from sudden unexpected infant death, forensic pathologist Dr. Roger Byard makes the following comment: "Lack of supervision at the time of fatal asphyxiation was a feature of all the cases where a history was available."[58]

Rather than suggesting parents should not bedshare, public health officials need to concentrate on providing access to information on how to maximize bedsharing safety, including information on what social and structural conditions can make bedsharing unsafe. It is unfortunate that certain medical institutions, hospitals and public health agencies seem unwilling to make distinctions between the act of cosleeping (including bedsharing) and the conditions within which it occurs. This unwillingness to make the distinction between safe and unsafe conditions suggests that health officials fail to appreciate, or choose not to acknowledge, the legitimate and special role mothers play in protecting their infants as they sleep next to them, or that mothers neither have the right nor the capability of doing so.

If you decide to cosleep or bedshare with your baby, you will no doubt encounter many parents, medical professionals, and media headlines that will try to convince you that you are not doing the best for your child. It is wise to remember that, above all else, **the only power that any of these groups or individuals have over you is what you choose to give them.** As long as the decision you make is an informed one, you can be confident that it is the right decision for you and your child.

PART II:

HOW TO COSLEEP

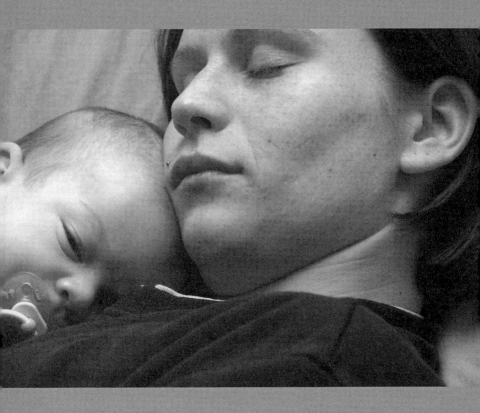

HOW TO SLEEP SAFELY WITH YOUR BABY

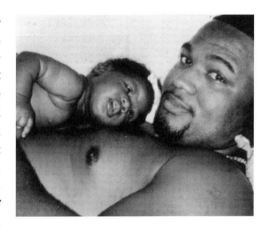

ach family has its own set of goals, needs and philosophies. While I suggest that all families should keep their infants sleeping in the same room with them if at all possible for at least the first six months or so, I don't feel that all families should bedshare. If you feel that you want the warmth, security, peace and nurturing that comes with bedsharing, then it is important to establish your cosleeping environment in a thoughtful and organized manner.

Let's start with the basics. I think it is appropriate for both parents who are in the bed to take responsibility, while asleep, for the baby being there. Just like those little signs attached to cars that say "Baby on Board," before you enter the bed where a baby will sleep next to you, think "Baby in Bed." You are responsible for knowing where your baby is and responding to that baby's presence. It takes a conscious decision to be responsive: just as you decide not to roll out of your bed, or may have decided that you WILL wake up early before your plane leaves, sleeping with a baby is more than a physical act, it is a mental act required by both parents in the bed even though one may be responding to the baby more frequently than the other.

Always lay your baby on his back, the natural position of every breastfeeding and cosleeping baby. Researchers have found that babies are at a ***much reduced risk*** of succumbing to SIDS if they sleep on their backs on a firm mattress with tight-fitting sheets, sleep with their faces unobstructed by pillows, blankets or stuffed animals, and sleep in a smoke-free setting.

If a mother smoked during her pregnancy, or smokes now, she should avoid bedsharing but have the baby sleeping next to her on a separate surface. If the father smokes, it is likewise best to have the baby sleep alongside the bed, rather than in the bed. As discussed in the next section, Peter Fleming's epidemiological study found that bedsharing with a smoking father raises risks to a problematic level.[59]

If routinely bedsharing, it is ideal to pull your bed away from walls and surrounding furniture into the center of the room, strip away the metal or wood framework, and lay the box spring on the floor with the mattress on top. As shown by the CPSC data, the most significant risks to a baby sleeping in a bed with an adult is not, as many assume, from an adult overlaying or rolling over onto the baby, but from the infant strangling or becoming wedged or trapped between a wall or a piece of furniture (like a bedside table) and a mattress, or between the bed frame, headboard or footboard and the mattress (see "The Consequences of Unsafe Cosleeping").

If you are unable or unwilling to pull your bed apart and place it in the center of a room, at the very least look for gaps and holes around your bed, and inspect the furniture and other objects which surround your mattress. Make sure no furniture is too close to the mattress, and be sure that your headboard, footboard and frame are tightly pressed to the mattress as well. Assume your baby will find a hole to fall into if one exists.

If you are breastfeeding and bedsharing remember to set the thermostat a bit lower as your own body next to the baby's acts to keep the baby warm; excessive warmth for an infant increases the chances of SIDS. Use hard, angular pillows, and keep them pushed away from the face of the infant. Light blankets are best, and little sleep suits might work well for your baby.

Careful considerations need to be made if either adult sleeping in the bed is obese. Excess weight might create a depression or space into which the baby may roll while sleeping. A particularly stiff mattress may compensate for this situation and no hard and fast rule about parental obesity and bedsharing can be empirically justified, except where no breastfeeding occurs AND other risk factors exist or predominate, in which case bedsharing should be avoided. These families can cosleep by placing the baby on a surface near the bed rather than in the bed itself. One study of the relationship between obesity and cosleeping (on a couch, a dangerous cosleeping environment for anyone) shows a tremendously elevated risk if couch cosleeping and obesity are present, although the data documents multiple independent risk factors, rather than one.[60]

Keep your baby away from duvets or heavy blankets that can flop over and cover the baby's face or nose, and be sure to keep other children out of your bed when your baby is sleeping in it.

Do not assume that pushing a mattress against a wall is safe because babies have become wedged in and suffocated **because the parents did not notice that the bed pulled away from the wall leaving just enough space into which a baby could fall and become asphyxiated.**

If you or your partner feel cramped in your bed, or if the bed is less than a full or queen size, then it is best not to bedshare. You should have enough room to spread apart.

The new folded mattresses appear to be not flat or stiff enough for maximum protection for your baby, so it is best to avoid sleeping with your baby on those particular mattresses. Never bedshare if you sleep on a waterbed.

One more note: when placing your baby down for a nap, use a spare walkie-talkie and monitor in the opposite way you use your primary one: turn the speakers around and broadcast the sounds and noises made in the active portion of the house into the room in which your baby is sleeping. This will provide background noise against which your baby can respond, enjoy arousals and otherwise sleep in a way that is the most natural for its body. Remember, at least 100 years of developmental science tells us that babies react much more healthfully to sound than to silence, especially if the sounds are human. Piping in voices is especially reassuring for infants and the voices represent a "life force" against which the baby's biology and physiology can respond. Turning the speakers around and feeding these sounds to the baby is proactive and protective, and can provide many of the same biological and developmental benefits for your baby that the act of cosleeping does.

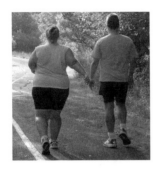

- If you are obese. Obese mothers are at much greater risk of overlaying their babies.

- If you smoked during your pregnancy.

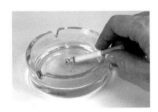

- If you, or your partner, smoke now.

- If you sleep on a waterbed, recliner, sofa, armchair, couch or bean bag.

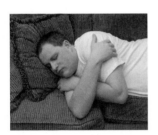

- If you sleep on multiple pillows, a sagging mattress, a feather mattress, or a sheepskin.

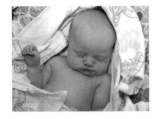

- If you use heavy bedding, such as comforters or duvets.

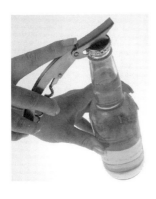

- In overheated rooms. Overheating is associated with higher rates of SIDS.

- If you, or another adult who will be sharing your bed, are under the influence of drugs or alcohol.

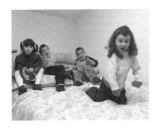

- If there are other children who can or are likely to climb into your bed.

- If there are pets who can or are likely to climb into your bed.

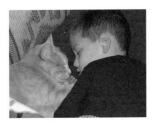

- If there are stuffed animals on the bed that could cover the baby's face.

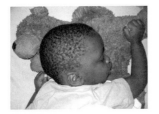

- If your baby is on her stomach. Babies should ALWAYS sleep on their backs.

THE CONSEQUENCES OF UNSAFE BEDSHARING

If you do not take proper precautions, this could happen to your baby:

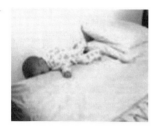

Entrapment between bed and wall.

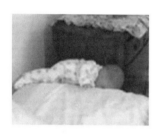

Entrapment between bed and object.

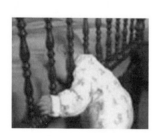

Entrapment in footboard of bed.

ALWAYS PRACTICE SAFE BEDSHARING!

COSLEEPING DO'S AND DON'TS

DO:

Make sure the baby is sleeping on a clean, firm, non-quilted surface. A mattress in the middle of the room without a frame is ideal.

Provide a smoke-free environment for your baby! If either parent smokes (no matter where you smoke), do not let your baby sleep in bed with you.

Place the baby on her back to sleep. If you breastfeed in bed, make sure the baby is on her back at the end of the feed.

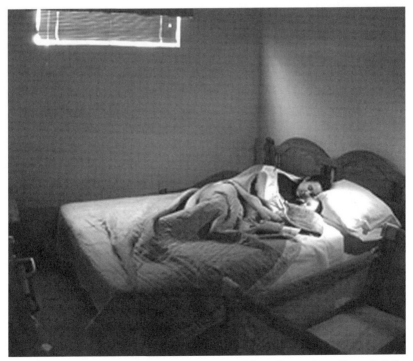

A realistic and safe cosleeping setup. Though the bed frame has not been dismantled, the mattress fits tightly against the headboard and the baby is not in a position where she might become trapped between the bed and the wall. A light blanket and only one pillow are being used.

DON'T:

Bedshare if either parent has consumed sedatives, medications, alcohol, or any substance that causes altered consciousness or marked drowsiness.

Bedshare if either parent is ill, tired to the point where it would be difficult to respond to the baby, or if either parent realizes that the primary caregiver is much more tired than usual.

Bedshare if there is any space between the bed and the wall where the baby could roll and become trapped. Make sure that the mattress fits tightly against the headboard and footboard and remove the bed frame if at all possible.

Bedshare if the parent sleeping next to the baby is markedly obese, unless the mother is breastfeeding and has considered how to compensate in some way for the greater weight differential.

Bedshare if older siblings who do not understand the risks of suffocation are sleeping in the same bed with infants less than one year old.

Bedshare if pets will be sharing the bed with the baby.

Place babies in an adult bed alone and unsupervised. **Never leave an infant alone on an adult bed.**

Use thick bedding. Sheets and blankets should be porous, preferably cotton. In cold weather, use layers of thin bedding rather than one heavier blanket.

Allow anything to cover the head or face of the baby.

Dress your baby too warmly—if you are comfortable, your baby probably is too. Remember that close bodily contact increases body temperature.

Leave long hair down or wear nightclothes with strings or ties. These pose a strangulation risk for the baby.

The Proper Way to Cosleep:

An idealized sketch of bedsharing when both parents do not smoke, are sober, have chosen to bedshare, and are breastfeeding their baby. The bed frame has been completely removed and the mattress has been placed at the center of the room away from walls and furniture. Light blankets and firm, square pillows are being used. No older children, pets, or stuffed animals are allowed in the bed.

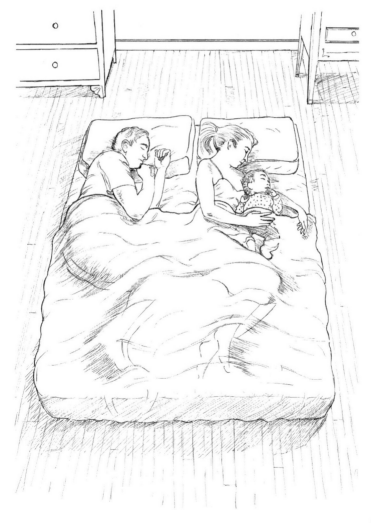

If You Choose To Bedshare...

While breastfeeding mothers are designed to sleep next to their babies, the furniture and bedding they use are not designed for infant use. This does not automatically mean bedsharing is unsafe, but it does suggest that extraordinary efforts are needed to maximize infant safety.

Bedsharing is complex. Unlike a crib environment that is designed for one small body, bedsharing is less socially and structurally stable. In some ways this is beneficial. A mother can and mostly does respond quickly if a baby moves to a dangerous place or into a dangerous position in the bed, or if the baby is making strange noises or no noises. As bedsharing rates have increased in Western countries such as Great Britain, Sweden, Australia and the United States, a disproportionately large number of infants are dying in adult beds. The overwhelming majority of these deaths are attributed to a particular risk factor associated with bedsharing, such as maternal smoking, prone infant sleep, drug use, sleeping with other children, or sleeping on pillows or in beds with gaps into which infants can fall and subsequently suffocate. A concerted awareness and a proactive approach designed to eliminate risk factors is essential, and the decision to bedshare must be made carefully.

If you choose to bedshare for any time during the night, it is crucial to your child's safety that you can anticipate possible threats. For example, how likely is it that a sibling or another adult will enter the bed? In such cases, these other bed sharers might not be as diligent as you are, or they might not have the capacity to protect the infant during sleep. Or, how likely is it that a family pet will jump on the bed, causing a rearrangement of blankets, pillows or bodies that inadvertently push the baby into harm's way? By assessing these risks, you can lessen the chance that your child will be in danger. You will be able to eliminate risk factors (such as by shutting the family pet away in another room) or, if these risks can't be avoided in your bed, you can place your baby on a separate sleep surface.

I cannot emphasize enough that most babies in the U.S. who die in adult beds become wedged between the mattress frame and a head- or footboard, between the mattress and a wall, or between the mattress and a nightstand. Unfortunately, there are more risk factors involved in bedsharing than there are in separate surface cosleeping situations. These risk factors must be identified and assessed by parents before they decide if and how they will share a bed with their baby.

If bedsharing is to be a routine, and if all other risk factors are eliminated, then the adult bed should be placed in the middle of the room, away from all walls or furniture. The mattress should be out of its frame and should be covered with simple, lightweight blankets, tight-fitting sheets and firm pillows. If other children enter the bed during the night, then babies might be better off cosleeping alongside the bed in a crib or bassinet.

Please remember, if you smoked during or after pregnancy, and if your baby is not exclusively breastfed, roomsharing is the safest form of cosleeping for your family.

If You Choose to Use a Cosleeping Product...

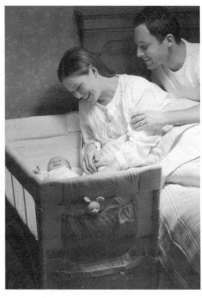

Since bedsharing is not an ideal sleep situation for all families, an excellent alternative is the use of a cosleeping device. These products come in many forms, including baskets that can be placed in the bed between parents, or separate sleep surfaces for babies that are connected to the parental bed. (It should be noted that no systematic tests have been completed on the safety of these devices. This does not necessarily mean that they are unsafe, just that they are untested.)

Devices that can be placed directly in the family bed provide a barrier for parents who fear that they might roll over onto their baby, or that their baby might fall off of the bed. They give mothers easy access for breastfeeding, and allow parents to be as close as possible to their baby while still offering some protection.

Cosleeping beds that can be attached to the parental bed are ideal for parents who are obese, regularly become intoxicated or over-tired, or who wish to continue using multiple pillows and comforters but still want to be close to their baby while they sleep. Because these devices have the baby sleep on a separate surface, parents can be comforted in knowing that the baby is safe from most dangers that are present in an adult bed.

Please see Appendix II for a list of available cosleeping devices.

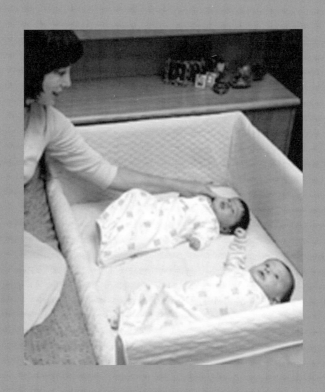

PART III:

FREQUENTLY ASKED QUESTIONS AND GENERAL ADVICE ABOUT COSLEEPING

HOW WILL COSLEEPING AFFECT MY RELATIONSHIP WITH MY PARTNER?

Every couple is different, but parenting is best done as a team with both parents fully committed to raising children in the same way. It is always best for parents or partners to discuss their goals, concerns, and philosophies and to strive toward a consensus, because whatever the challenges might be, they are easier solved if you both agree on what experiences all of you want to share.

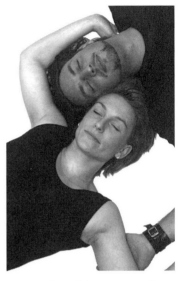

If both partners agree, bedsharing or roomsharing can be a wonderful way for Dad to spend time with the baby, talking, stroking and (if bedsharing) enjoying skin-to-skin contact. Especially if Dad is separate from the baby many hours during the day, bedsharing can be an important way to keep fathers emotionally involved.

Most popular parenting books on infant sleeping arrangements seem to ignore mentioning the ways in which practices can vary in meaning and function from one family to another. I want you to be aware that **no experience is the same for any two families because all families are different.**

That said, many parents wonder how cosleeping will affect their own relationship. Because your baby and your family are unique, it is impossible to say with certainty how cosleeping will affect your relationship. But we can say the following: new parents are faced with numerous challenges and rewards as they adjust to their roles as mothers and fathers, and developing a sleeping pattern that works for your family is just one challenge among many.

There are several things to keep in mind as you develop your cosleeping patterns.

Cosleeping doesn't have to affect tenderness and closeness between spouses. With the baby in bed, you can still talk, touch, laugh, massage and otherwise enjoy the connection with your partner. Intimacy will have to be less spontaneous. You may need to start scheduling time together when someone else can tend to the baby, find some other place to be intimate after the baby falls asleep, or move the baby into a crib or bassinet after he falls asleep.

Learn about child development. Kids go through lots of different transitions as they grow, and each stage is just a stage. Parenting with your partner will be easier—and less frustrating—if you understand what is going on developmentally with your baby. Whether it is teething, separation anxiety, nighttime fears, or something else, these are all stages—and they are all temporary.

WILL COSLEEPING GET IN THE WAY OF MY CHILD'S ABILITY TO BE INDEPENDENT?

Ultimately, absolutely not, but it may delay your baby's willingness to be alone when she sleeps. Sometimes parents are under the mistaken impression that if they don't train their babies to sleep by themselves, somehow some developmental or social skill later in life will be kept from them, or they worry that their babies will never exhibit good sleep patterns as adults. In reality, there has never been a scientific study anywhere that has shown any benefit whatsoever to sleeping through the night at young ages, or even sleeping through the night as adults.

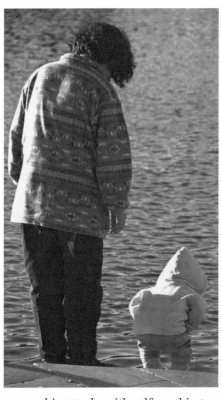

Independence and autonomy have nothing to do with self-soothing or forcing babies to learn how to sleep by themselves. Studies have shown recently that children who routinely sleep with their parents actually become more independent socially and psychologically, and are able to be alone better. The idea that you shouldn't pick up a baby or touch a baby during the night, which is believed by many who promote solitary sleep, is completely antithetical to a hundred years of biological information on what constitutes good development: the development of empathy, the development of autonomy, the ability to be alone when you need to be alone, and the ability to interrelate and to become interdependent with others. As you begin to know your child better and identify your priorities as a parent, you will guide your child toward these goals. When compared to solitary sleeping children, children who have coslept tend to make friends easily, are more innovative, better able to control their tempers, and are better problem-solvers.[61, 62, 63, 64]

Earlier we talked about parenting trade-offs, and this is an important and useful concept here. For example, should you choose to routinely cosleep all night every night with your child, you should be prepared for the possibility that, when you are ready to wean your child from your bed, they may not be on the same timetable as you. One study found that, compared with solitary sleepers from birth, infants who cosleep from birth either learn or accept sleeping alone about a year later than infants who have no choice but to sleep alone. So the trade off may be this: the emergence of independent solitary sleeping in children may be delayed with routine cosleeping, but eventually separate sleep will not be a problem for your child, and the good news is that as parents you derived great feelings and memories from cosleeping. Along with those experiences, your child may have developed a more permanent capacity for self-sufficiency, resilience, comfort with affection, and the ability to be alone when necessary.[65]

WILL WE BE ABLE TO GET A GOOD NIGHT'S REST IF WE BRING OUR BABY INTO OUR BED?

The answer to this question depends in part on exactly how parents define a "good night's sleep," and whether bedsharing is a choice made by the parents or a situation they feel was imposed on them by their child's inability to sleep alone. But remember that the reason that many families unexpectedly decide to bedshare is that it permits the family to get more sleep. It is more accurate to say that some parents, while still happy with their decision to bedshare for emotional reasons, are not able to get as much uninterrupted sleep.

For many families it remains worth it to bedshare with older children, even if on some nights Dad or Mom makes a hasty retreat to an empty bed somewhere else in the house for some extra rest they feel they need—a system I refer to as "musical beds." Sometimes one parent takes the call from a child sleeping in another room and enters the child's bed, stays for while, then slips back into their own bed. Moms and Dads often take turns—or maybe just Dad does the nighttime

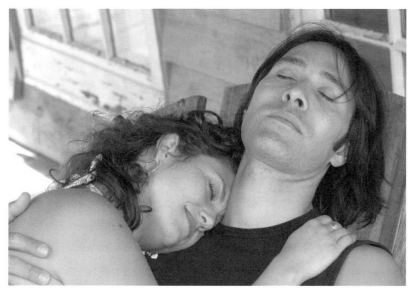

responding (as I did). For families that like this method, it can work very well. (Upon reflection, I can honestly say I think back with gratitude for those times when my son called me into his bed to snuggle upon waking and feeling a bit insecure.) Again, each family should work to find what arrangements work best for them.

Contrary to popular belief, and according to the mothers themselves, the choice to bedshare with infants tends to promote a longer, more restful night's sleep for both babies and parents alike, and this is especially true if the mother is breastfeeding. A baby sleeping in a separate room, in order to elicit a feeding from the mother, needs to cry. This generally makes the baby less calm and more excited, even before the breastfeeding begins. While bedsharing mothers may have many more arousals, they perceive that their sleep is better when they are sleeping with their babies. And, of course, if you do experience difficulty sleeping with your child in your bed, you can still experience many of the benefits of cosleeping by having your baby sleep on a separate surface in the same room.

MANY PEDIATRICIANS SAY I WILL CREATE A "BAD HABIT" THAT WILL BE HARD TO BREAK IF I BEDSHARE. IS THIS TRUE?

This ubiquitous warning is based on subjective, perceived values, not science. One family's "bad habit" is another family's most treasured time together. And for most (though maybe not all), bedsharing feels pretty darn good, and for all the right reasons. Like adults, infants and children will be reluctant to give up something that feels right to them. That said, any human habit can be broken and the way new sleeping arrangements are introduced depends on who the parents and children are and the special characteristics of the family.

There is absolutely nothing wrong with deciding that you are ready to have your child sleep in his or her own room, but the trick is to trust your own knowledge of your child in deciding how best to do this. Methods tried by some parents include making bedtime full of stories and rituals unique to your child or offering a sleeping companion doll or favorite object, easing the child from the bed by having the child

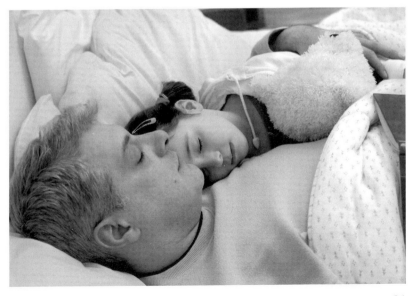

sleep on the floor or a mat next to the bed or on a cot or bed in the room but not in the bed, or merely stressing the excitement of a new room or having special privileges for an older child. Changing routines is a necessary part of growing up, and the transition away from cosleeping can be a positive experience for your child.

WHAT ABOUT NAPTIMES?

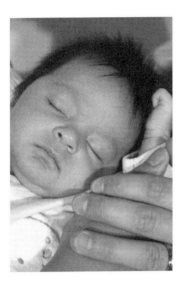

Most babies do not mind sleeping alone during naps during the day—it is the darkness of nighttime that is intimidating. But it is ideal to not isolate babies even for naps.

Try to let your baby nap in a bassinet or crib wherever there are people around, if this is possible. Don't worry about your baby not being able to fall asleep, because most babies can sleep in the middle of a rock concert when they are tired. The old idea of "Shhhh! ... the baby is sleeping," only conditions a baby to sleep lightly and to stir at each extraneous noise. Babies feel secure hearing the voices of their brothers or sisters and parents while sleeping. The level of normal noises in a household assures a level of arousal in your baby that's probably just about right for the safest possible sleep.

And remember to purchase an extra set of baby monitors and put the speaker next to your baby! (See page 63.)

IF I HAVE TWINS OR MULTIPLES, SHOULD WE COSLEEP?

As with any aspect of caring for twins, there are added challenges to bedsharing, especially without the proactive involvement of your partner or spouse. My general recommendation is to place at least one twin back in the crib or bassinet after feeding and sleeping with one twin or multiple at a time, to place both or all infants back in the same crib or bassinet to cobed with each other (see the next chapter), or to place two or more bassinets next to each other.

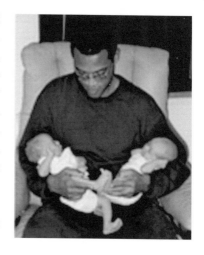

If you do not have the kind of spouse or partner that sees him or herself as an active partner in the care of your twins, it is best not to fall asleep with the twins in the bed. Moreover, if regularly bedsharing with your twins, it is essential to have a king-size bed and a partner who is more than a passive participant, and who has agreed to work with you to take responsibility for knowing exactly where each twin is at all times.

If the second adult does not agree to take responsibility for at least one twin, but you want to continue to bedshare, then do not leave one twin between yourself and your partner, but rather have both twins in front of you so that you can curve your body around them and shield them from your bed-mate.

Keeping yourself and your twins at some distances from each other will be important too, only because it is easier for one twin to want to snuggle as close to you, and in the process, as close (perhaps too close) to his sibling as he can get. Use only the lightest of blankets to ensure free air passage for both twins. Being mindful of the fact that hungry infants are quite capable of mistaking a sibling's nose for a breast is worth preparing for, because as strange or as funny as it may seem, one twin sucking on the nose of the other can quickly dehydrate the other. Yes, it has happened.

I recommend that if there is a partner in the bed who has no interest in monitoring or taking responsibility for one or both twins, after each breastfeed (and if not breastfeeding at all), it is best to place the infants back in a bassinet or crib to cobed. (Karen Gromada has written a wonderful book on parenting multiples.)[66]

WHAT IS COBEDDING? DOES IT SERVE THE SAME PURPOSE AS BEDSHARING?

From a scientific point of view, this is an area that is little investigated. The term for cosleeping twins is "cobedding." Cobedding is another form of cosleeping, and is very different from what the majority of this book has been concerned with. Cobedding takes the form of two bodies of equal 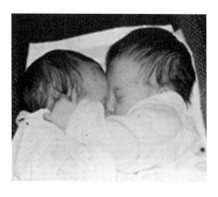 size and weight in the same crib. How cobedding functions, and its role in infant development and safety, is very different from other forms of cosleeping. Since twins and multiples in general (for reasons still unknown) are associated with a higher risk for SIDS, questions pertaining to what kind of sleep environment might best protect them or put them at increased risk is especially critical. Questions pertaining to cobedding emerge against the larger background of trying to understand why premature births occur, as many twins are born premature. Prematurity is the leading cause of hospitalization during the neonatal period, and is responsible for up to 75% of neonatal illness and deaths, so this is an area in need of much further exploration.[67]

The challenge of all newborns in making their way from the womb to the worldly environment is to re-establish some kind of "biorhythmic balance" by stabilizing the functions of sleep-wake cycles, eating patterns, blood chemistry levels, and respiratory and heart rates. Two teams of researchers have argued that the mutual sensory exchanges that are facilitated by cobedding may enhance the ability of any one twin to accomplish this task specifically by improving breathing, using energy more efficiently and, in general, reducing the twins' stress levels. It is known, for example, that the stress response which leads to increased cortisol production can negatively impact growth and development and generally alter thermal regulation, sleep duration, breathing and heart rate in potentially negative ways. These researchers found that, similar to what is observed to occur in the womb, cobedded twins move close together, touch and suck on each other, hold each other, and hug one another. Studies done by Dr. Helen Ball show that twins smile at each other and are often awake at the same time, supporting several anecdotal reports by parents of twins that their own infants prefer to be together, and that their babies settle better together and sleep more soundly when cobedded. Given the challenges of caring for two babies, as Dr. Ball points out from her studies, it is not surprising that parents will come to practice any behavioral care pattern which tends to maximize their own sleep and ease the burden of caring for and feeding two babies simultaneously.[68, 69, 70]

Nowadays when you hear a recommendation against cobedding, it often illustrates cultural biases against cosleeping in general where medical authorities assume—without any data—that if some instances of bedsharing between an adult and a baby are dangerous, then certainly two infants of equal body size must likewise pose a mutual threat. When and where there is a gap in our knowledge, or little information is available, recommendations (whether medical or not) quickly rely on generalizations, stereotypes, and anecdotal information, which is then passed on as if proven scientifically to be true. In this case, studies of bedsharing involving adults and infants are being applied to the question of whether or not it is safe or beneficial for twins to share a crib. Some hospital nursery wards are already assuming that the AAP's recommendation against bedsharing applies to twins when, in fact, no twin studies were considered as the basis for those SIDS guidelines and no evidence-based considerations have, thus far, been used to justify hospital policies that argue against cobedding.

COBEDDING ARRANGEMENTS

As the following drawings from Dr. Ball's study of 60 parents of twins shows, there are many different ways that parents of twins arrange a cobedding sleep environment for their infants:

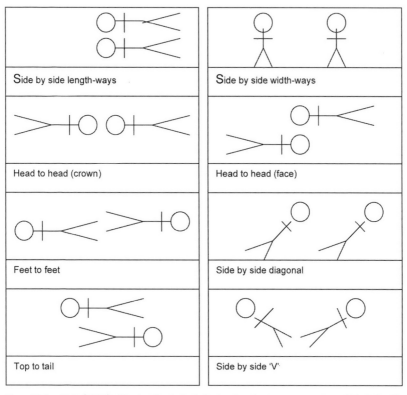

Side by side length-ways	Side by side width-ways
Head to head (crown)	Head to head (face)
Feet to feet	Side by side diagonal
Top to tail	Side by side 'V'

From Helen Ball (2006): "Caring for twin infants: sleeping arrangements and their implications." Evidence-Based Midwifery 4 (1) :10-16. Courtesy of: Evidence-Based Midwifery.

IS THERE ANYTHING DIFFERENT ABOUT COSLEEPING WITH AN ADOPTED BABY?

Depending on their ages and experiences, adopted infants and children may have heightened needs for affection and contact, but, if older, they may not be used to intimacy. Watch carefully how your child reacts to you and respond accordingly. It is also helpful, where possible, to know your child's history of experiences and assess what special needs or processes may be required to integrate the child into your family and to establish secure, safe and trustworthy new relationships.

If you have adopted an infant and not a child, of course, there is no difference. Regardless of cultural origin, place of birth, or ethnicity, all babies have the same needs. Since attachment between any of us can be greatly enhanced by contact, cosleeping behavior can greatly facilitate the developing bond between your adopted child and yourself. It may be the case that adoption agencies require infants or children to have their own rooms. But you will be joining millions of parents whose nighttime care and associations with their children are hardly defined nor limited by the number of bedrooms they have, or where a crib may be located.

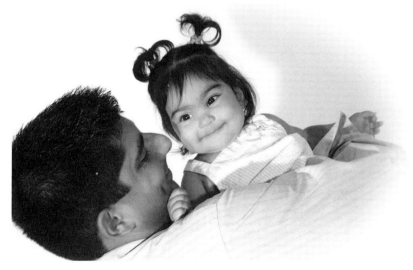

WHAT SHOULD A COSLEEPING FAMILY KNOW ABOUT TRAVELING TOGETHER?

During the first few years of life, you will find your infant or child will feel especially reassured sleeping in your company when away from home. Many parents permit cosleeping while traveling who do not ordinarily practice it.

There does seem to be an elevated risk of SIDS for babies who experience a previously unknown sleep environment. That is, babies between 2 and 4 months of age who are left to sleep alone while traveling and who ordinarily do not sleep alone have an increased risk (however slight) of dying from SIDS. And the reverse seems also to be true. A baby who does not ordinarily bedshare but who does while sleeping away from its home is at an increased risk of SIDS because she is in a new sleep environment. The bottom line: perhaps it is best while traveling to mimic as closely as possible what you ordinarily do at home. If you bedshare, bedshare; if you sleep apart, sleep apart.

Keep in mind that if you are bedsharing while traveling, you need to ensure that the bedsharing setup is safe for your baby (see Part II: How to Cosleep). **When you are traveling or on vacation, risk factors that may endanger your baby are still present. Risks may, in fact, be increased, so it will pay to be extra careful as to where and how your baby is sleeping while traveling.**

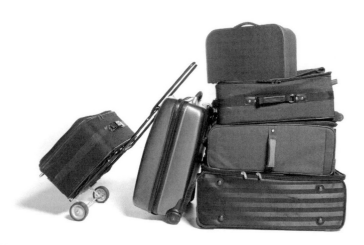

WILL MY CHILD BE DIFFERENT, IN ANY NEGATIVE SENSE, IF I CHOOSE TO COSLEEP OR BEDSHARE?

O!

Sleeping arrangements never, by themselves, create any specific kind of relationship that has not already been shaped by what occurs during the day. Sleeping arrangements only reflect the nature of the relationship a parent and child already share before they come to bed. In other words, sleeping arrangements generally reflect and sometimes strengthen, contribute to, or exaggerate the nature of the relationship that already exists, whether good or bad.

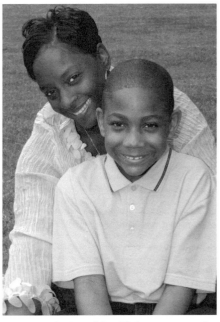

Sleeping arrangements do not create a relationship: if the nature of a relationship is very, very good during the day, cosleeping simply makes whatever is already good just as good or even better at night.

In contrast, if a parent is depressed or is resentful of the infant during the day, these same dynamics will impact the child negatively during the night if the parents choose to cosleep. That said, cosleeping can be a wonderful way for content and affectionate parents to continue to deepen the bond with their child during the night.

HOW LONG SHOULD I COSLEEP WITH MY CHILD?

However long you want to! In fact, how long an infant or child sleeps in proximity to her parents has never been a concern throughout all of the evolution of our species. As long as cosleeping is enjoyed by everyone involved and the relationship it reflects is healthy during the day, 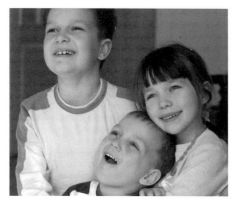 cosleeping in some form or another never has to stop...but, of course, it will. There is no specific cut-off after which suddenly, or even gradually, the family cosleeping arrangement becomes harmful, unless someone in the arrangement is no longer pleased or at some point the situation has became socially, psychologically or physically unhealthy or undesired by a participating member of the family. Cosleeping (whether bedsharing or roomsharing) could never be best if all participants do not feel comfortable with the practice, and this is always the best time to stop. If anyone involved does not wish to cosleep, then cosleeping should never be forced.

I am reminded of the number of times my South American undergraduate students sheepishly come up to me after my lectures on cosleeping to whisper their stories that they could never tell to their peers for fear of ridicule. More often than not, they wish to tell me they STILL cosleep with their parents when they return home for the holidays! One of my young friends described how all of the kids jump into their parents' bed for conversation, storytelling, eating, watching TV, and for the simple enjoyment of sleeping together and being with each other in their parents' bed.

SHOULD WE COSLEEP IF MY PARTNER IS NOT THE BABY'S FATHER?

There is one study that has shown an increased risk of an infant dying when bedsharing with an unrelated adult male or other adult. However, the group that was studied for the most part had more than one risk factor present when these babies died.[71] My guess is that if an unrelated sleeping partner is committed to an infant, assumes responsibility for her, considers the bedsharing infant his or her responsibility in the same ways the mother does, then the bedsharing should be as safe as it would be if the bio-

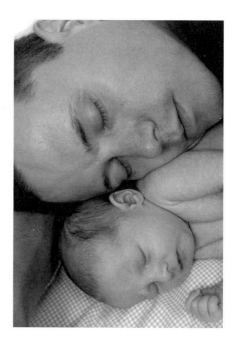

logical father or an adoptive parent were bedsharing. But the point is worth repeating. Unrelated adults may not care to be responsible for the infant in the same way as a biological or adoptive parent might be, or may choose to disregard their own responsibility for the infant's safety. In any situation in which this is true, I would recommend against bedsharing. Instead, place the baby next to the bed on a different surface.

WHAT LONG-TERM EFFECTS WILL MY BABY EXPERIENCE IF WE COSLEEP?

It has never been proven, nor shown, nor is it even probable, that sleeping with your baby has any kind of negative long-term effects when the relationships between those involved are healthy. Instead, experts are finding that cosleeping can help develop positive qualities, such as more comfort with physical affection, more confidence in one's own sexual gender identity, a more positive and optimistic attitude about life, or more innovativeness as a toddler and an increased ability to be alone. One major epidemiological study showed cosleeping school-age children as being under-represented in psychiatric populations. And, while I do not know if you might regard this as a blessing or a curse, a survey of college-age subjects found that males who coslept with their parents between birth and five years of age had significantly higher self-esteem, experienced less guilt and anxiety, and even reported greater frequency of sex! Cosleeping is part of a loving, supportive environment that parents produce for their children, and this, in turn, will give them the confidence to grow into social, happy, loving adults.[72]

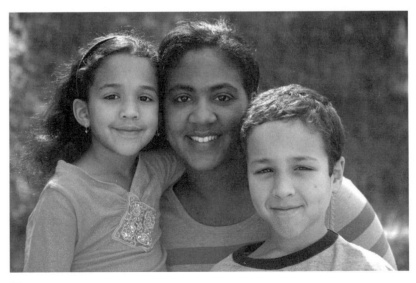

IS IT POSSIBLE TO REDUCE NIGHT FEEDINGS IN A COSLEEPING SITUATION?

It is a difficult and unique process to wean a baby who has slept next to you from birth. The decision to wean is important, and should only be made if you feel it is necessary.

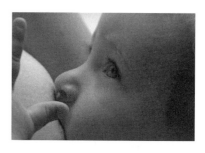

Some babies might have difficulty adjusting to less breastfeeding. One strategy for less night breastfeeding is to breastfeed your baby more during the day. Placing a barrier between your breast and the baby, or sleeping facing in opposite directions can sometimes reduce the infant's detection of milk nearby and eliminate some feeds, as can simply placing the baby in a crib in your room, or next to you in a bassinet.

If your baby is crying to be fed, Dad can walk with the baby to help her learn a new association. Dad's role in weaning a baby from night feedings can be very rewarding for fathers, leading to a new aspect of the attachment relationship with the baby.

Trusting and using your own judgment and experience with your baby is important—and every baby will give you different insights as to what might work best for them and only them. Like the decision to cosleep or bedshare, the decision to wean has to be made carefully and with full attention to the needs of each individual family.

SHOULD I BEDSHARE WITH MY PREMATURE OR UNDERWEIGHT BABY?

In almost all of the epidemiological studies of which I am aware, infants who are small for gestational age or premature are disproportionately represented as SIDS victims and as victims of sudden unexpected infant death in bedsharing situations. While the reasons for this are not yet known, and could possibly include in-utero developmental events or assaults to the fetal nervous system (some of which are induced by maternal smoking, which can cause intra-uterine growth retardation), it is probably safer not to bedshare with your underweight or premature infant. Routine bedsharing does not seem to be found to contribute to the survival of these more fragile infants, so it is best avoided. Place your premature or underweight baby right next to your bed on a different surface, but not in bed with you. Skin-to-skin contact while awake, however, is extremely protective, and sensory exchanges with an adult are known to be clinically beneficial to developmentally disadvantaged infants. The more holding, carrying and breastmilk made available for these special babies, and the more physical interactions you have with them, the better.

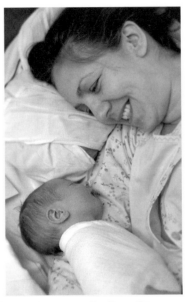

Appendices

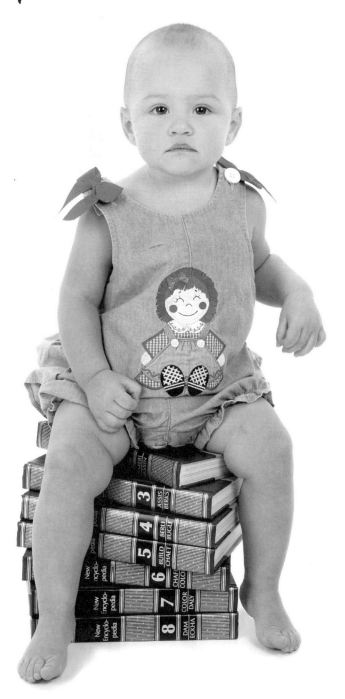

APPENDIX I

BEDSHARING RESOURCES AND FURTHER READING

Books/Periodicals

Fleiss, Paul M. *Sweet Dreams: A Pediatrician's Secrets for your Child's Good Night's Sleep.* December, 2000. ISBN: 737304944

Most new parents quickly and sadly discover the difficulty of getting a child first to go to sleep, and then to sleep throughout the night. Dr. Fleiss, a noted family pediatrician for more than 30 years, shares his secrets for discovering a child's natural sleep patterns, developing positive bedtime rituals, nutritional and lifestyle aids to sleep, and how cosleeping affects normal growth and development.

Goodavage, Maria and Jay Gordon, M.D. *Good Nights: The Happy Parents' Guide to the Family Bed.* June, 2002. ISBN: 312275188

Good Nights puts your concerns about the family bed to rest, with fun and easy-to-use guidance on safety, coping with criticism, and even keeping the spark in your marriage (albeit outside the bedroom). With warmth and humor, Dr. Jay Gordon, a nationally-recognized pediatrician who has endorsed the family bed for decades, and Maria Goodavage, a former *USA Today* staff writer with training in sleep research, give you everything you'll need in order to thrive—and at times, simply survive—with the family bed.

Jackson, Deborah. *Three in a Bed: The Benefits of Sharing Your Bed with Your Baby.* August, 1999. ISBN: 158234051

This classic book details the invaluable benefits for breastfeeding mothers, reviews the history of babies in the bed and, through interviews with parents, explores current attitudes to the idea. It also contains a new perspective on the tragedy of cot death, as well as practical advice on how to sustain your sex life, hints on safety in the bed and answers to common objections.

Mothering Magazine Special Edition, No. 114. September/October 2002.

An entire issue of the magazine for natural parenting devoted to the issue of cosleeping. Go to http://www.mothering.com/ to order back copies of the 40-page issue for $8.

Sears, Martha & William Sears. *How to Get Your Baby to Sleep.* July, 2002. ISBN: 316776203

Dr. Bill and Martha Sears share their expertise on developing a nighttime routine, creating a safe sleep environment for your child, how to dress your baby for sleep, how to avoid SIDS, helping your child unwind at bedtime, the benefits of sleep-sharing, determining how much sleep your child needs, coping with a light sleeper or an early riser, and tips for getting your toddler to stay in bed.

Sears, William. *Nighttime Parenting: How to Get your Baby and Child to Sleep.* November, 1999. ISBN: 452281482

Written to make that job easier and to help the whole family—mother, father, baby—sleep better, this book helps parents understand why babies sleep differently than adults, offers solutions to nighttime problems, and even describes how certain styles of nighttime parenting can aid in child spacing and lower the risks of SIDS.

Sunderland, Margot. *Science of Parenting: Practical Guidance on Sleep, Crying, Play and Building Emotional Wellbeing for Life.* May, 2006. ISBN: 0756618800

Based on over 700 scientific studies into children's development, child psychotherapist Dr. Margot Sunderland explains a hands-on parenting approach that helps children to realize their full potential.

Thevenin, Tine. *Family Bed.* February, 2002. ISBN: 039952729X

An "excellent" (Jane Goodall, Ph.D.) guide to the pros and cons of having children sleep in their parents' beds.

DVDs / Videos

Ball, Dr. Helen, Sally Inch and Marion Copeland. *The Benefits of Bedsharing.* 2005. Available from Platypus Media. www.PlatypusMedia.com

This warm and instructional video/DVD, based on research at the Mother-Baby Sleep Lab at the University of Durham (UK) as well as sleep research from around the world, is an accurate and sensible guide to the benefits and safety issues of bedsharing

Websites

UNICEF UK Baby Friendly Initiative leaflet on bedsharing

http://www.babyfriendly.org.uk/parents/sharingbed.asp

A leaflet with information on the benefits and risks of bedsharing, designed to help parents make informed decisions about safely sharing a bed with their babies. Downloads available in English, French, Spanish and Portuguese.

James J. McKenna and the University of Notre Dame's Mother-Baby Behavioral Sleep Laboratory

http://www.nd.edu/~jmckenn1/lab/

Author James J. McKenna's official website, full of further information on cosleeping and bedsharing.

Dr. Helen Ball and the Durham University Parent-Infant Sleep Laboratory

http://www.dur.ac.uk/sleep.lab/

A United Kingdom-based parent-child sleep study center, with lots of information.

Dr. William Sears

http://www.askdrsears.com

The official website of the grandfather of the attachment parenting movement, Dr. William Sears, his wife and registered nurse Martha, and two of their sons, both pediatricians.

Organizations

Academy of Breastfeeding Medicine is a worldwide organization of physicians dedicated to the promotion, protection and support of breastfeeding and human lactation. By uniting members of various medical specialties with this common goal, ABM is developing clinical protocols for managing common medical problems that may impact breastfeeding success.

140 Huguenot Street, 3rd floor
New Rochelle, NY 10801
800-990-4226
ABM@bfmed.org
http://www.bfmed.org/

American SIDS Institute is a national nonprofit health care organization dedicated to the prevention of sudden infant death and the promotion of infant health through aggressive, comprehensive nationwide programs.

509 Augusta Drive
Marietta, GA 30067
770-426-8746
prevent@sids.org
http://www.sids.org/

Attachment Parenting International networks with parents, professionals and like-minded organizations around the world. In addition to providing assistance in forming Attachment Parenting support groups, API functions as a clearinghouse providing educational materials, research information, consultative, referral and speaker services to promote Attachment Parenting concepts.

2906 Berry Hill Drive
Nashville, TN 37204
615-298-4334
info@attachmentparenting.org
http://www.attachmentparenting.org

International Lactation Consultant Association is the professional association for International Board Certified Lactation Consultants (IBCLCs) and other health care professionals who care for breastfeeding families. Their vision is a worldwide network of lactation professionals, and their mission is to advance the profession of lactation consulting worldwide through leadership, advocacy, professional development, and research.

1500 Sunday Drive, Suite 102
Raleigh, NC 27607
919-861-5577
info@ilca.org
http://www.ilca.org

La Leche League International is an organization founded in 1956 by seven women who wanted to make breastfeeding easier and more rewarding for both mother and child. The organization offers information and encouragement—primarily through personal help—to women who want to breastfeed their babies. Their mission is to help mothers worldwide to breastfeed through mother-to-mother support, education, information, and encouragement and to promote a better understanding of breastfeeding as an important element in the healthy development of the baby and mother.

1400 N. Meacham Road
Schaumburg, IL 60173-4808
847-519-7730
llli@llli.org
http://www.llli.org

United States Breastfeeding Committee is a collaborative partnership of organizations. The mission of the committee is to protect, promote and support breastfeeding in the U.S. The USBC exists to assure the rightful place of breastfeeding in society.

2025 M Street NW, Suite 800
Washington DC 20036
202-367-1132
info@usbreastfeeding.org
http://www.usbreastfeeding.org

APPENDIX III

COSLEEPING PRODUCTS

COSLEEPER® BEDSIDE SLEEPER (ORIGINAL) BY ARM'S REACH

The Arm's Reach® CO-SLEEPER® bassinet is one of the most useful attachment tools. It allows parents and babies to have their own bed space, yet stay within touching distance of each other.

In addition to allowing for bonding between parents and baby, nighttime feedings are made easier when parents sleep within arm's reach of baby. Sleeping close to their infant allows parents to make up for missed time during the day and to connect with their baby at night.

Besides being extremely well designed and sturdily constructed, the CO-SLEEPER® bassinet converts to additional uses and that makes it an economical investment. The ORIGINAL model can convert to a play yard. They are also portable, having their own bag for traveling and easy storage.

There are different models, sizes, colors, and prints available to better coordinate with your bedroom.

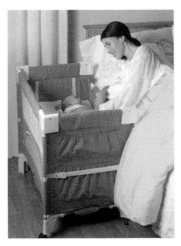

For more information, visit www.armsreach.com or call 800-954-9353 or 805-278-2559.

BABY BUNK BY SIDE BY SIDE SLEEPING, INC.

For nursing moms, the Baby Bunk™ infant sleeper is an ideal arrangement, and for moms who decide to bottle feed, the sleeper lets you spend your nights together, helping to keep you closely bonded, but giving you each your own space.

For information, call or fax at 800-697-8944, send an e-mail to Ilene@babybunk.com, or visit www.babybunk.com.

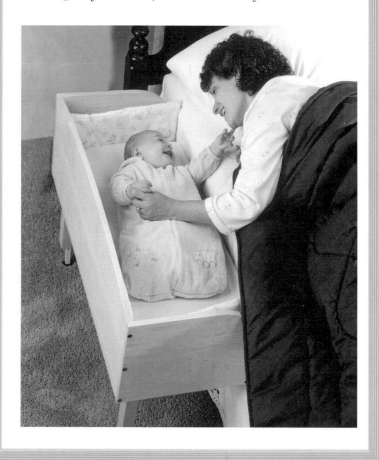

HUMANITY FAMILY SLEEPER & CO-SLEEPING BEAN BY HUMANITY INFANT AND HERBAL

The bed top sleeper makes bedsharing a breeze!

This simple but superb product keeps baby safe from rolling off the bed as well as protecting the bedding from mishaps. It is practical, portable and provides years of protection, as well as the best night's sleep for cosleeping mothers and babies.

For more information, please call 207-221-5318, or visit www.humanityinfantandherbal.com.

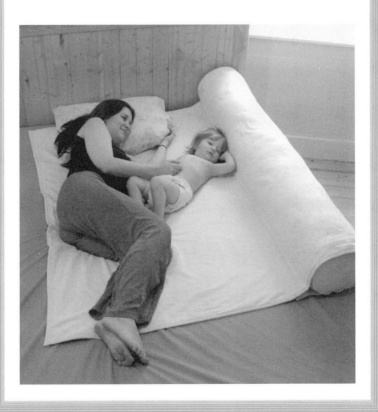

SNUGGLE NEST, BY BABY DELIGHT, INC.

The Snuggle Nest is placed between the parents' pillows, thus removing the infant from the "rollover zone," where infants might get rolled on or overheated from parents' bodies and bedding, and it has a rigid plastic tray with three strong walls that serve to block adult pillows and bedding from baby's face, and also fill the gap between the adult mattress and the headboard.

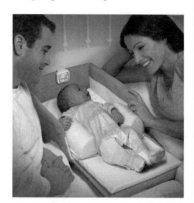

For retailers, please call toll-free 877-810-9350, or visit www.BabyDelight.com.

The Nursing Nest by Peaceful Pea

The Nursing Nest® is the product that (aside from being a useful tool to help protect Baby from accidental parental rollover while bonding, breastfeeding or co-sleeping in the family bed), allows Mom to Table Top breastfeed so she may keep her baby at her breast for several hours at a time while she stays on top of her daily schedule.

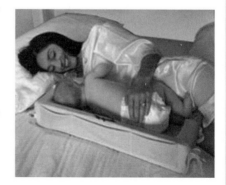

For more information, call 310-514-9112 or visit www.peacefulpea.com.

APPENDIX III

SUMMARY OF AMERICAN ACADEMY OF PEDIATRICS (AAP) SUDDEN INFANT DEATH (SIDS) POLICY STATEMENT: NOVEMBER 1, 2005

In the fall of 2005, the American Academy of Pediatrics released a policy statement on Sudden Infant Death Syndrome, revising their previous statement from March 1, 2000. This statement included a review of recent studies on SIDS, and issued recommendations. A summary of the statement follows:

> There has been a major decrease in the incidence of sudden infant death syndrome (SIDS) since the American Academy of Pediatrics (AAP) released its recommendation in 1992 that infants be placed down for sleep in a nonprone [abdomen facing away from sleep surface] position. Although the SIDS rate continues to fall, some of the recent decrease of the last several years may be a result of coding shifts to other causes of unexpected infant deaths. Since the AAP published its last statement on SIDS in 2000, several issues have become relevant, including the significant risk of the side sleeping position; the AAP no longer recognizes side sleeping as a reasonable alternative to fully supine [abdomen facing away from sleep surface] sleeping. The AAP also stresses the need to avoid redundant soft bedding and soft objects in the infant's sleeping environment, the hazards of adults sleeping with an infant in the same bed, the SIDS risk reduction associated with having infants sleep in the same room as adults and with using pacifiers at the time of sleep, the importance of educating secondary caregivers and neonatology practitioners on the importance of "back to sleep," and strategies to reduce the incidence of positional plagiocephaly associated with supine positioning.

The AAP's recommendations included the following controversial advice:

A separate but proximate sleeping environment is recommended: The risk of SIDS has been shown to be reduced when the infant sleeps in the same room as the mother. A crib, bassinet, or cradle that conforms to the safety standards of the Consumer Product Safety Commission (CPSC) and ASTM (formerly the American Society for Testing and Materials) is recommended. "Cosleepers" (infant beds that attach to the mother's bed) provide easy access for the mother to the infant, especially for breastfeeding, but safety standards for these devices have not yet been established by the Consumer Product Safety Commission.

Although bed-sharing rates are increasing in the United States for a number of reasons, including facilitation of breastfeeding, the task force concludes that the evidence is growing that bed sharing, as practiced in the United States and other Western countries, is more hazardous than the infant sleeping on a separate sleep surface and, therefore, recommends that infants not bed share during sleep. Infants may be brought into bed for nursing or comforting but should be returned to their own crib or bassinet when the parent is ready to return to sleep.

Consider offering a pacifier at nap time and bedtime: Although the mechanism is not known, the reduced risk of SIDS associated with pacifier use during sleep is compelling, and the evidence that pacifier use inhibits breastfeeding or causes later dental complications is not. Until evidence dictates otherwise, the task force recommends use of a pacifier throughout the first year of life..."

The full statement can be found at:
> http://aappolicy.aappublications.org/cgi/content/full
> /pediatrics;116/5/1245

For further information, contact:
> The American Academy of Pediatrics
> 141 Northwest Point Boulevard
> Elk Grove Village, IL 60007-1098
> 847-434-4000
> http://www.aap.org

A number of renowned and respected parenting educators and organizations responded to this report. A sampling of their statements are reprinted in the following appendices.

Appendix IV

DR. JAMES MCKENNA'S THOUGHTS ON THE AMERICAN ACADEMY OF PEDIATRICS' RECOMMENDATIONS ON BEDSHARING—MAY 2007

What exactly is the AAP position on bedsharing? What groups support bedsharing as a legitimate choice and how is it that bedsharing seems to come out looking so bad in public conversations that include the media?

Put simply, the American Academy of Pediatrics, in their 2005 recommendation (see Appendix III), describes bedsharing as being "hazardous" and associated with increasing the chances of an infant dying either from SIDS or from some kind of "sudden unexpected death." Following a year-long review of case control epidemiological studies (unfortunately no other studies were included), the sub-committee on infant sleep position and SIDS, after further consultations with other ad hoc experts (Drs. Bradley Thach and James Kemp of Washington University in St. Louis and myself), recommended that babies ought to be removed from the parents' bed when the parents return to sleep. The committee accepts the idea that while asleep a mother is unable to safely interact or respond to the infant's needs, to assure the infant's safety either from some form of overlying or suffocation caused by her own nearness, or by the mattress, bedding materials or structures, or some combination of these.

On the positive side, this same committee recommended that to help avoid SIDS infants should, of course, sleep on their backs and not on their stomachs or sides, since too many babies who died from SIDS began their sleep on their sides but rolled onto their stomachs and died. And for the first time, the committee recommended that infants should not sleep alone in a room by themselves but rather in a room with a committed adult caregiver—that is, infants should roomshare. The committee also argues that breastfeeding should be encouraged. One could say, then, that while the AAP recommends against bedsharing, it recommends cosleeping in the form of "proximate" separate surface cosleeping. This is a somewhat radical proposition given our cultural history, but is based on the fact that babies sleeping alone in a room by themselves have at least a 25-50 % greater chance of dying from SIDS, according to three epidemiological studies.

I think it is fair to generalize that most pediatricians know nothing more about SIDS than what the general summaries of SIDS research written in the pediatric newsletters report. Unless a physician slept with his or her own parents as a child, or enjoyed sleeping with his or her own infant, there is a very good chance that they will accept the AAP opinions that bedsharing is dangerous and increases the chances of suffocation or SIDS. It should be reassuring to know also that many other scientists, including myself, who have studied SIDS and other aspects of human infant and maternal biology for a very long time, disagree with the AAP's unqualified recommendation against bedsharing—not because there are many instances in which bedsharing should be recommended against, but because one negative recommendation against all bedsharing is too simplistic and scientifically flawed.

For more information on Dr. Jim McKenna's research and publications, visit his webpage at: http://www.nd.edu/~jmckenn1/lab

APPENDIX V

UNITED STATES BREASTFEEDING COMMITTEE (USBC) STATEMENT IN RESPONSE TO AAP: OCTOBER 17, 2005

Mixed Credibility of the Revised AAP SIDS Prevention Recommendations

The American Academy of Pediatrics (AAP) released revised recommendations for Sudden Infant Death Syndrome (SIDS) prevention last week, one of which provides valuable new information to help parents protect their infant, while others not only lack a solid scientific basis but also entail some risks.

The AAP now recommends that infants sleep in the same room as their parents because this is associated with a reduced risk of SIDS. While studies have consistently found that isolating infants for sleep (in a separate bedroom) is associated with a higher risk of SIDS, this information has not previously been widely disseminated. Sleeping near one's infant has also been shown to increase maternal responsiveness to the infant's nighttime physiologic signals and to make it easier for mother to succeed with breastfeeding. Breastfeeding, in turn, is linked to a reduced risk of many acute and chronic illnesses, including a 21% lower all-cause infant mortality rate in an analysis by the National Institutes of Health, and to a reduced risk of SIDS in a number of studies.

Two recommendations in the new AAP statement have stirred particular concern: to give babies pacifiers and to remove the infant from the parental bed prior to sleep. Both recommendations are problematic in a number of ways, including that they lack a clear scientific basis, constrain parental choice, complicate the potentially challenging process of putting infants to sleep, and impair breastfeeding.

Because early pacifier use reduces breastfeeding duration, the AAP SIDS statement recommends waiting until one month of age (to allow breastfeeding to get off to a good start) before starting pacifiers in breastfed infants. Even beyond this period pacifiers entail health risks, however, and may undermine breastfeeding success.

A number of studies (but not all) have found an association between pacifier use and lower rates of SIDS. But these studies cannot determine if the relationship is causal, and therefore whether pacifier use can reduce the risk of SIDS. Nevertheless, even if the oral stimulation of sucking were protective, only those infants lacking the natural source of nighttime suckling, breastfeeding, would be likely to benefit from an artificial pacifier source of such stimulation. Only in such "at risk" groups might it make sense to assume the health risks of pacifier use which include yeast infections, oral malocclusion, and ear infections.

Data are also lacking to justify telling parents whether or not they should sleep with their infants—beyond informing them of the protective effect of sleeping in the same room as their baby. In the best controlled studies, infant safety is not associated with whether the baby sleeps in the parents' bed per se, but on specific environmental factors that warrant attention whether the baby is in a bed, a crib, or other sleeping surface. For example, SIDS has been associated with prone sleep position, maternal smoking, soft mattresses, and bedding near the baby that could cover the head. Avoidable exceptions in which bedsharing itself has been associated with an increased risk of SIDS include the use of particularly unsafe furniture (e.g., couches, which are associated with a 25-fold increased risk of SIDS) and parent smoking or incapacitation due to alcohol or drug use, or exhaustion.

The United States Breastfeeding Committee recommends caution before advising pacifiers for breastfeeding infants even after one month of age. It also emphasizes the importance of closeness to one's infant and supports the statement of the Section on Breastfeeding of the AAP that mother and infant sleep in close proximity.

The USBC is a national committee made up of over 30 organizations that protect, promote, and support breastfeeding.

Footnotes can be viewed at: www.usbreastfeeding.org.

The USBC is an organization of organizations. Opinions expressed by the USBC are not necessarily the position of all member organizations and opinions expressed by USBC representatives are not necessarily the position of the USBC.

United States Breastfeeding Committee
2025 M Street, NW Suite 800
Washington DC 20036
202-367-1132
Fax: 202-367-2132
office@usbreastfeeding.org
http://www.usbreastfeeding.org

APPENDIX VI

LA LECHE LEAGUE INTERNATIONAL (LLLI) STATEMENT IN RESPONSE TO AAP: OCTOBER, 2005

Schaumburg, IL—La Leche League International (LLLI) is concerned about the October 10, 2005 policy statement on Sudden Infant Death Syndrome (SIDS) issued by the American Academy of Pediatrics (AAP) Task Force on SIDS. The recommendations about pacifiers and cosleeping in the statement reflect a lack of basic understanding about breastfeeding management.

Pacifiers, which are recommended in this policy statement, are artificial substitutes for what the breast does naturally. Breastfed babies often nurse to sleep for naps and bedtime. The recommended pacifier usage could cause a reduction in milk supply due to reduced stimulation of the breasts and may affect breastfeeding duration.

LLLI recognizes that safe cosleeping facilitates breastfeeding. One important way cosleeping can help a mother's milk supply is by encouraging regular and frequent feeding. Well-known research on safe cosleeping practices by Dr. James McKenna, Director of the Mother-Baby Behavioral Sleep Laboratory at Notre Dame University was disregarded by the task force.

Also, the obvious omission of input by the AAP's Section on Breastfeeding may account for the fact that breastfeeding management issues were not taken into consideration. Dr. Nancy Wight, President of the Academy of Breastfeeding Medicine, comments that this statement "represents a truly astounding triumph of ethnocentric assumptions over common sense and medical research." Dr. Wight also states, "There are many physician members of the AAP who do not agree with these recommendations."

Although the authors do state that breastfeeding is beneficial and should be promoted, their recommendations about pacifier use and cosleeping could have a negative impact on a mother's efforts to breastfeed. The statement causes confusion for parents and falls seriously short of being a useful and comprehensive policy.

LLLI, a non-profit organization that helps mothers learn about breastfeeding, has an international Professional Advisory Board. The LLLI Center for Breastfeeding Information is one of the world's largest libraries of information on breastfeeding, human lactation, and related topics. Monthly meetings are offered to pregnant women and nursing mothers and babies to learn about breastfeeding management.

La Leche League International
1400 N. Meacham Road
Schaumburg, IL 60173-4808
847-519-7730
Toll-free: 800-LA-LECHE
Fax: 847-519-0035
llli@llli.org
http://www.lalecheleague.org

APPENDIX VIII

INTERNATIONAL LACTATION CONSULTANTS ASSOCIATION (ILCA) STATEMENT IN RESPONSE TO AAP: NOVEMBER 28, 2005

The sudden unexpected death of an otherwise healthy infant is a tragedy no family should have to experience. In an effort to continue to reduce rates of sudden infant death syndrome (SIDS*) in the United States, the American Academy of Pediatrics Task Force on SIDS has issued a revised set of recommendations that have provoked controversy because of their potential impact on breastfeeding families.[1] Specifically, concerns about the new recommendations to increase the use of pacifiers and to discourage bed sharing have been raised by the Academy of Breastfeeding Medicine, as well as other breastfeeding advocacy groups.[2-4] Because these recommendations will be used to determine standards of practice among physicians, it is important that lactation consultants understand their basis and significance for breastfeeding families.

The International Lactation Consultant Association (ILCA) recognizes that much of the controversy surrounding the recommendations results from inconsistency in research findings related to breastfeeding and pacifier use, bed-sharing/co-sleeping and SIDS. Inconsistent results in breastfeeding related research often occur due to lack of a clear definition of breastfeeding.[5] Comparing children who were "never" breastfed to those who were "ever" breastfed combines highly varied practices into the same groups, potentially mixing children who breastfed once in the hospital with those who exclusively breastfed for several months. Well-designed research trials should define both exclusivity and duration of breastfeeding.[5] Very few of the studies cited in the AAP policy statement defined either exclusivity or duration. The baby who is exclusively breastfed for 6 months is the appropriate reference model.[6,7]

There have been many studies examining the association between pacifier use and breastfeeding duration among both term and preterm infants. Many of the observational studies indicate that pacifier use, at any stage of lactation, is associated with reduced breastfeeding exclusivity or duration.[8-18] However, randomized controlled trials indicate that pacifier use, after the first month postpartum, is not significantly associated with shorter breastfeeding duration.[19-21] It is possible that pacifier use is an indicator for breastfeeding difficulties rather than a cause of problems or that other factors contribute to both pacifier use and early weaning. On the basis of the evidence from the randomized trials examining the association between pacifier use and reduced risk for SIDS,[22] the AAP committee recommended that pacifiers be avoided by breastfeeding families in the first month postpartum to ensure that breastfeeding is well established. Lactation consultants will play an important role in ensuring that pacifier use after the first month does not interfere with successful lactation.

ILCA applauds the AAP for recommending sleeping in close proximity to one's infant to reduce risk of SIDS. Advising against any bed-sharing for the breastfed infant is highly controversial.[7,23] The breastfed infant is more likely to sleep supine and suckle frequently through the night, naturally achieving the potentially SIDS reducing goals of less deep sleep and frequent brief arousals. Given the need for night feeds in the early months postpartum, bed-sharing is used as a means by parents to reduce the time they spend awake during the night. In a study of over 10,000 families, breastfeeding parents were 3 times more likely than bottle-feeding parents to bed-share.[24] The potential effects of the guidelines on breastfeeding duration and exclusivity have yet to be explored. It is important that lactation consultants educate themselves about all the options for sleeping arrangements for families and to follow-up on any breastfeeding-related concerns.

ILCA continues to recommend exclusive breastfeeding for 6 months followed by the addition of complementary, age-appropriate solids and continued breastfeeding for 2 years and beyond. In keeping with the new AAP guidelines:

Pacifiers should be avoided until breastfeeding is well established.

Mothers who are having difficulty with breastfeeding should be closely monitored, particularly if they choose to use pacifiers.

Infants should sleep in close proximity to their mothers though not necessarily in the same bed.

Further research is needed on the sleeping practices of healthy infants and the association between co-sleeping and infant feeding patterns.

Infants should never sleep with other children, with parents who smoke or abuse drugs or alcohol, on couches or other locations where entrapment might occur.

Infants should always be placed on their backs to sleep, on a firm mattress without any pillows or other soft, loose bedding.

Community education efforts should focus strongly on increasing exclusive breastfeeding for the first 6 months of life, decreasing parental smoking and smoking during pregnancy and educating parents, non-parental caregivers and hospital staff about the dangers of non-supine sleep positions for infants.

While the new guidelines remain controversial, the recommendations to avoid pacifiers in the first month and encourage parents to sleep in the same room with their infants are positive steps toward the promotion of breastfeeding. Lactation consultants must continue to call for research in these important areas of SIDS prevention. As the evidence-base grows, it will be the responsibility of the AAP to refine their guidelines in line with research outcomes.

The International Lactation Consultant Association is a worldwide network of lactation professionals. For more information on increasing exclusive breastfeeding, see ILCA's Clinical Guidelines for the Establishment of Exclusive Breastfeeding published in 2005, available at: www.ilca.org.

*The term SIDS also refers to sudden unexplained infant death (SUID).

Footnotes can be viewed at: www.ilca.org

International Lactation Consultant Association
1500 Sunday Drive, Suite 102
Raleigh, NC 27607
919-861-5577
Fax: 919-787-4916
info@ilca.org
http://ww.ilca.org

REFERENCES

1. McKenna, James J., Mosko, Sarah, Dungy, Claiborne and McAninch, Jan. (1990). "Sleep and Arousal Patterns of Co-Sleeping Human Mother-Infant Pairs: A Preliminary Physiological Study with Implications for the Study of the Sudden Infant Death Syndrome (SIDS)." *American Journal of Physical Anthropology, 82(3)*: 331–347.

2. Mosko, Sarah, McKenna, James J., et al. (1993). "Infant-Parent Co-sleeping: The Appropriate Context for the Study of Infant Sleep and Implications for SIDS." *Journal of Behavioral Medicine, 16(6)*: 589–610.

3. Keller, M.A. and W.A. Goldberg (2004). "Co-sleeping: Help or hindrance for young children's independence?" *Infant and Child Development*: 369–388. DOI:10.1002/icd.365.

4. Mosko, S., Richard, C., & McKenna, J. (1997). "Maternal sleep and arousals during bedsharing with infants." *Sleep, 20(2)*: 142–150.

5. Nelson, E.A.S et al. (2001). "International Child Care Study: Infant Sleeping Environment." *Early Human Development. 62*: 43–55.

6. McKenna, J. J., Thoman, E. B., Anders, T. F., Sadeh, A., Schechtman, V. L., & Glotzbach, S. F. (1993). "Infant-parent co-sleeping in an evolutionary perspective: implications for understanding infant sleep development and the sudden infant death syndrome." *Sleep, 16(3)*: 263–282.

7. McKenna, James J. and L.Volpe. "An Internet Based Study of Infant Sleeping Arrangements and Parental Perceptions." *Infant Behavior and Child Development* special issue on cosleeping. Wendy Goldberg, Editor.

8. Montagu, Ashley Touch. (1986). "The Significance of Human Skin."(3rd edition). Harper Row: New York.

9. Field, T. M. (1998). "Touch therapy effects on development." *International Journal of Behavioral Development, 22*: 779–797.

10. Field, T. (2001). "Massage therapy facilitates weight gain in preterm infants." *Current Directions in Psychological Science, 10*: 51–54.

11. Whiting, J. W. M. (1981). "Environmental constraints on infant care practices." *Handbook of Cross-Cultural Human Development*. R. H. Munroe, R. L. Munroe, R. L. and B. B. Whiting, editors. New York: Garland STPM Press.

12. Field, T. M., Schanberg, S. M., Scafidi, F., Bauer, C. R., Vega-Lahr, N., Garcia, R. et al. (1986). "Tactile/kinesthetic stimulation effects on preterm neonates." *Pediatrics, 77*: 654–658.

13. Montagu, Ashley Touch. (1986). *The Significance of Human Skin* (3rd edition). Harper Row: New York.

14. Brazy, J. E. (1988). "Effects of crying on cerebral blood volume and cytochrome aa3." *The Journal of Pediatrics, 112*: 457–461.

15. "Controlled Crying." (2002). Australian Association of Infant Mental Health Position Paper.

16. Reiter, M. and Field, T. (1985). "The Psychobiology of Attachment and Separation." New York; Academic Press.

17. Mosko, S., Richard, C., and McKenna, J. (1997a). "Infant arousals during mother–infant bed sharing: Implications for infant sleep and sudden infant death syndrome research." *Pediatrics, 100*: 841–849.

18. Anderson, G. C. (1995). "Touch and the kangaroo care method." In T. M. Field (Ed.), *Touch in early development*, Mahwah, NJ: Lawrence Erlbaum: 33–51.

19. Ball, Helen. (2003) Breast Feeding, bedsharing and infant sleep. Birth. *Issues in Prenatal Care, 30(3)*:181–188.

20. Ludington-Hoe, S. et al. (1999). "Birth-related fatigue in 34–36-week preterm neonates: rapid recovery with very early kangaroo (skin-to-skin) care." *Journal of Obstetric, Gynecologic, and Neonatal Nursing, 28(1)*: 94–103.

21. de Chateau, P. W., B. (1977). "Long-term effect on mother-infant behaviour of extra contact during the first hour post partum. II. A follow-up at three months." *Acta Paediatr Scand, 66(2)*: 145–151.

22. DiPietro, J., Larson, S.K., Porges, S.W. (1987). "Behavioral and heart rate pattern differences between breast fed and bottle fed neonates." *Developmental Psychology, 23(4)*: 467–474.

23. Widstrom, A. et al (1990). "Short term effects of early suckling and touch of the nipple on maternal behaviour." *Early Human Development, 21*: (153–163).

24. Vial-Courmont, M. (2000). "The kangaroo ward." *Med Wieku Rozwoj* 4(2 suppl 3) : 105–17.

25. Stewart, M.W., Stewart, L.A. (1991). "Modification of sleep respiratory patterns by auditory stimulation: indications of techniques for preventing sudden infant death syndrome." *Sleep, 14(3)*: 241–8.

26. Thoman, E.B. and Graham, S.E. (1986). "Self-regulation of stimulation by premature infants." *Pediatrics, 78*: 855–60.

27. Mosko, S., Richard, C., McKenna, J., Drummond, S., & Mukai, D. (1997). "Maternal proximity and infant CO2 environment during bedsharing and possible implications for SIDS research." *American Journal of Physical Anthropology, 103(3)*: 315–328.

28. American Academy of Pediatrics Section on Breastfeeding. (2005). "Breastfeeding and the use of human milk." *Pediatrics, 115*: 496–506.

29. R. Carpenter, L. Irgens, P. Blair, P. England, P. Fleming, J. Huber, G. Jorch, P. Schreuder. "Sudden unexplained infant death in 20 regions in Europe: case control study." *The Lancet, 363(9404)*: 185–191.

30. Quillin, S. I. M., and Glenn, L. L. (2004). "Interaction between feeding method and co-sleeping on maternal-newborn sleep." *Journal of Obstetric, Gynecologic, and Neonatal Nursing, 33*: 580–588.

31. American Academy of Pediatrics Section on Breastfeeding. (2005). "Breastfeeding and the use of human milk." *Pediatrics, 115*: 496–506.

32. Konner, M. & Worthman, C. (1980). "Nursing frequency, gonadal function, and birth spacing among !Kung hunter-gatherers." *Science, 207*: 788–791.

33. McKenna, J. J., Mosko, S.S., et al. (1997). "Bedsharing promotes breastfeeding." *Pediatrics, 100*: 214–219.

34. Ball, H.L. (2003). "Breastfeeding, bed-sharing and infant sleep." *Birth, 30(3)*: 181–188.

35. Dewey, K.G. (1998). "Growth characteristics of breast-fed compared to formula-fed infants." *Biol Neonate, 74*: 94–105.

36. Ball, H. L. (2002). "Reasons to bed-share: why parents sleep with their infants." *Journal of Reproductive and Infant Psychology, 20(4)*: 207–221.

37. Chen, A., Rogan, W. (2004). "Breast feeding and the risk of post-neonatal death in the United States." *Pediatrics, 113*: E435–E439.

38. Lucas, A., Morley, R. et al. (1992). "Breast milk and subsequent intelligence quotient in children born preterm." *Lancet, 339*: 261–264.

39. Newcombe, P.A. et al. (1994). "Lactation and reduced risk of premenopausal breast cancer." *New England Journal of Medicine, 330(2)*: 81–87.

40. Ainsworth, M.D.S., Blehar, M.C., Waters, E., Wall, S. (1978). "Patterns of attachment: A psychological study of the strange situation." Hillsdale, NJ: Lawrence Erlbaum.

41. Posada, G., Jacobs, A., Richmond, M.K., Carbonell, O.A., Alzate, G., Bustamante, M.A., et al. (2002) "Maternal caregiving and infant security in two cultures." *Developmental Psychology, 38*: 67–78.

42. Thompson, R.A. (1999). "Early Attachment and later development". J. Cassidy & P.R. Shave (Eds.). New York: Guilford Press. *Handbook of attachment: Theory, research and clinical applications:* 265–286.

43. Ball, H. Ball, Helen L. (2006). "Parent-Infant Bed-sharing Behavior: effects of feeding type, and presence of father." *Human Nature: an interdisciplinary biosocial perspective 17(3)*: 301–316.

44. Ball, H. L. (2002b). "Reasons to bed-share: why parents sleep with their infants." *Journal of Reproductive and Infant Psychology, 20(4)*: 207–221.

45. Anisfeld, E., Casper, V., Nozyce, M., and Cunningham, N. (1990). "Does infant carrying promote attachment? An experimental study of the effects of increased physical contact on the development of attachment." *Child Development, 61*: 1617–1627.

46. Rigda, R.S., et al. "Bed sharing patterns in a cohort of Australian infants during the first six months after birth." *Journal of Pediatrics and Child Health, 36(2)*: 117–121.

47. Ball, H. L. (2002b). "Reasons to bed-share: why parents sleep with their infants." *Journal of Reproductive and Infant Psychology, 20(4)*: 207–221.

48. National Sleep Foundation (2005). Sleep in America Poll. Retrieved 6/28/06 http://www. sleepfoundation.org/_content/hottopics/2005 _summary_of_findings.pdf.

49. McKenna, James J. and L.Volpe. "An Internet Based Study of Infant Sleeping Arrangements and Parental Perceptions." *Infant Behavior and Child Development* special issue on cosleeping. Wendy Goldberg , Editor.

50. Ball, H. Ball, Helen L. (2006). "Parent-Infant Bed-sharing Behavior: effects of feeding type, and presence of father." *Human Nature: an interdisciplinary biosocial perspective, 17(3)*: 301–316.

51. McKenna, James J. and Thomas McDade. "Why Babies Should Never Sleep Alone: A Review of the Cosleeping Controversy In Relationship To SIDS, Breast Feeding and Bedsharing." *Pediatric Respiratory Reviews, 6*: 134–152.

52. Spock, B. (1988). Dr. Spock on parenting: Sensible advice from America's most trusted child-care expert. (M. Stein, Ed.). Pocket Books: New York.

53. National Sleep Foundation (2005). Sleep in America Poll. Retrieved 6/28/06 http://www.sleepfoundation.org/_content/ho ttopics/2005_summary_of_findings.pdf.

54. Ferber, Richard. (2006). "Solve Your Child's Sleep Problems" Fireside: London and New York.

55. Nakamura, S., Wind, M., and Danello, M. (1999). "Review of hazards associated with children placed in adult beds." *Archives of*

Pediatric and Adolescent Medicine, 153(10): 1018–23.

56. Fleming, P., Blair P. and McKenna, J.J. (2006). "New knowledge, new insights and new recommendations" *Arch. Dis. Child, 91:* 799–801.

57. McGarvey, C. and McDonnell, M. (2006). "An eight year study of risk factors for SIDS: bedsharing vs. non-bedsharing." *Arch Dis. Child, 91:* 318–323.

58. Byard, R. , Beal,S, Bourne A(1994). Potentially dangerous sleeping environments and accidental asphyxia ininfancy and early chioldhod. *Arch. Dis in Children, 71:* 497–500.

59. Fleming, P., Blair, P., Bacon, C., et al. (1996). "Environments of infants during sleep and the risk of the sudden infant death syndrome: Results of 1993–1995 case control study for confidential inquiry into stillbirths and deaths in infancy." *British Medical Journal, 313:* 191–195.

60. Carroll-Pankhurst, C. and Mortimer, A. (2001). "Sudden infant death syndrome, bedsharing, parental weight, and age at death." *Pediatrics, 107(3):* 530–536.

61. Heron, P. (1994). "Non-Reactive Cosleeping and Child Behavior: Getting a Good Night's Sleep All Night, Every Night," Master's thesis, Department of Psychology, University of Bristol.

62. Crawford, M. (1994). "Parenting Practices in the Basque Country: Implications of Infant and Childhood Sleeping Location for Personality Development." *Ethos* 22, no. 1: 42–82.

63. Lewis, R.J. and Janda L.H. (1998). "The Relationship between Adult Sexual Adjustment and Childhood Experience regarding Exposure to Nudity, Sleeping in the Parental Bed, and Parental Attitudes toward Sexuality." *Archives of Sexual Behavior, 17:* 349–363.

64. Forbes, J.F. et al. (1992). "The Cosleeping Habits of Military Children." *Military Medicine, 157:* 196–200.

65. Keller, M.A. and Goldberg, W.A. (2004). "Cosleeping: Help or hindrance for young children's independence?" Infant and Child Development, 13: 369–388. DOI:10.1002/icd.365.

66. Gromada, Karen and Gromada-Kerkoff. (2006). Mothering Multiples: Breast Feeding and Caring For Twins.

67. Lutes, L. and Altimer, L. (2001). "Co-bedding multiples." *Newborn and nursing reviews 1(4).* Available online at http://www.nainr.com/scripts /om.dll/serv.

68. Nyqvist, K.H. and Lutes, L.M. (1998). "Co-bedding twins: a developmentally supportive care strategy." *Journal of Obstetrical, Gynecological, and Neonatal Nursing, 27(4):* 450–56.

69. Ball, Helen. (2006). "Caring for twins: sleeping arrangements and their implications" *Evidence Based Midwifery, 4(1):* 10–16.

70. Ball, Helen. "Together or Apart? A behavioral and physiological investigation of sleeping arrangements for twin babies." Midwifery in press.

71. Hauck, F. R. et al. (2003). "Sleep environment and the risk of sudden infant death syndrome in an urban population." The Chicago Infant Mortality Study. *Pediatrics, 111 (5):* 1207–1214.

72. McKenna, James J. (2000). "Cultural influences on infant and childhood sleep biology and the science that studies it: Toward a more inclusive paradigm. Sleep and Breathing In Children and Pediatrics." J Laughlin, C, Marcos, J. Carroll (Eds). Marcel-Dekker Pub: 99–130.

INDEX

About Platypus Media®

Platypus Media is an independent publisher dedicated to promoting family life by creating and distributing high quality materials about families. We strive to be the premier source of products that have a broad appeal to families and the professionals who work with them. We celebrate the importance of family closeness to the full and healthy development of children. Our goal is to bring materials to the market that parents love, children enjoy, teachers appreciate, and parenting professionals value.

Platypus Media currently offers a selection of books, booklets, videos, DVDs, plush toys, T-shirts and other products, many of which have garnered widespread praise. As the well-respected pediatrician, Dr. William Sears, says: **Platypus Media's books not only promote literacy, they promote families!** We hope you will find as much pleasure in them as we have had in creating and bringing them to you!

For more information about our publications, bulk purchasing, or to contact us for a catalog, visit us at PlatypusMedia.com.

Platypus Media,® LLC
627 A Street, NE
Washington, DC 20002
Toll-free: 1–877–PLATYPS (1–877–872–8977)
    or 202–546–1674
Fax: 202–546–2356
www.PlatypusMedia.com
Info@PlatypusMedia.com

Platypus media

Books for
parents, teachers
and parenting
professionals

Platypus Media® is committed to the promotion and protection of breastfeeding. We donate six percent of our profits to breastfeeding organizations.

Bulk Ordering Information

Agencies and organizations may receive a bulk discount for quantity orders. Please contact us at the address above or email us at Info@PlatypusMedia.com.

NOW AVAILABLE FROM PLATYPUS MEDIA

The Benefits of Bedsharing

A well–researched, accurate, and sensible guide to the benefits and safety issues of bedsharing.

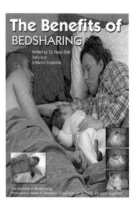

Bedsharing can help the whole family feel good and be better rested. Most breastfeeding mothers around the world sleep with their babies, yet modern beds are designed for adult comfort, not infant safety. When the baby is sleeping separately from the mother, Mother responds to her baby's needs in minutes; if they are bedsharing, she responds in seconds—thus there is less disruption to everyone's sleep. *The Benefits of Bedsharing* features a variety of mothers and fathers cosleeping at home, as well as in hospital environments. Examples of risky situations reinforce the importance of creating a safe bedsharing environment. The DVD includes the same program as the VHS plus full chapter navigation, slide show, and a still frame library...excellent for parent trainers and child care professionals.

The Benefits of Bedsharing *is an accurate, scientifically based presentation of how to bedshare safely with baby. With excellent narration and graphical representations, this DVD summarizes the worldwide research findings, revealing distinct advantages for breastfeeding mothers who bedshare, and includes specific descriptions and pictures of what is safe and what is not. Talk about Evidence-Based Medicine, it doesn't get any better than this!*

James J. McKenna, Ph.D.

Finally, a video that provides clear information on the benefits of bedsharing with our children. This has been the way of raising children for thousands of years, and now we get to choose it, too!

Jan Tritten, founder and editor, *Midwifery Today*

The Benefits of Bedsharing
Dr. Helen Ball, Sally Inch and Marion Copeland
Running time: 12 minutes
2005
VHS $80 / DVD $125

Breastfeeding Facts for Fathers

Breastfeeding is considered a woman's issue, yet research shows that the father's stated preference for breastfeeding was found to be the most important factor influencing a woman's decision to breastfeed. Conventional wisdom has it that breastfeeding excludes men, but the reality is that men have a crucial role to play in not only encouraging any individual woman to breastfeed, but also in helping to create a culture in which breastfeeding women are visible, accepted and valued.

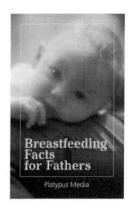

This upbeat pamphlet gives a man the information he needs to support not only his partner's breastfeeding, but breastfeeding in general, and addresses a new father's typical concerns about breastfeeding.

With contributions by:

- Lawrence M. Gartner, MD, Chair, AAP Work Group on Breastfeeding
- Jack Newman, MD, author, University of Toronto
- William Sears, MD, author, University of Southern California
- James J. McKenna, Ph.D., author, University of Notre Dame
- Brian Palmer, DDS, consultant for hospital sleep centers

Expectant fathers want to provide the best for their families. When they understand and support breastfeeding that is exactly what they are doing. Kudos to Platypus Media for making Breastfeeding Facts for Fathers as entertaining as it is informative.

David Meyers, MD, Georgetown University Medical Center

Breastfeeding Facts for Fathers is a fact-packed and fun-filled book for new dads. Questions about the mysterious world of breastmilk are answered with precision and panache. This booklet is a must-have for obstetricians, pediatricians, midwives and new parents.

Milton Werthmann, Jr., MD, Neonatologist and Pediatrician

8 1/2" x 5 1/2", 24 pages
Full–color cover, black & white interior
Photographs, illustrations and tables
Soft cover, stapled, $5.95
ISBN 1–930775–12–1/978–930775–12–1

Breastfeeding At a Glance: Facts, Figures and Trivia About Lactation

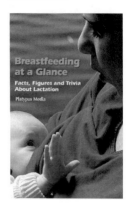

Dia L. Michels and Cynthia Good Mojab, MS with Naomi Bromberg Bar-Yam, PhD

This handy booklet is attractive, fascinating and succinct!

It answers frequently-asked questions about breastfeeding; lists benefits for the mother, baby and community; provides breastfeeding rates; information on mammal lactation, breastfeeding and the law; a resource list and more. Includes more than 20 charts, tables and illustrations. Fully referenced.

A fact-filled breastfeeding overview in an accessible format!

8 1/2" x 5 1/2", 24 pages
Full-color cover, black & white interior
Photographs, illustrations and tables
Softcover, stapled, $5.95
ISBN 1-930775-05-9 / 978-1-930775-05-3

I don't go anywhere without my copy of Breastfeeding at a Glance! *As a person who speaks to the press on a daily basis, I rely on materials that are thorough, factual, and meaningful. The authors answer the questions people want to know about breastfeeding, but what makes this little book invaluable is that every section is fully referenced. Anyone who wants to speak with authority on lactation needs a copy of this book!*

Mary Lofton, Director of Public Relations
La Leche League International

Make it a set—buy *Breastfeeding at a Glance* with *Breastfeeding Facts for Fathers* for just $9.99. A great deal for a wealth of breastfeeding information!

Breastfeeding Booklet Set:
1-930775-25-3/978-1-930775-25-1